D1605946

HANDBOOK *of*
CORONARY STENTS

HANDBOOK *of*
CORONARY STENTS

Fourth Edition

Edited by

Patrick W Serruys MD PhD FACC FESC
Professor of Interventional Cardiology
Erasmus University
Head, Department of Interventional Cardiology
Heart Centre
University Hospital Rotterdam-Dijkzigt
Rotterdam
The Netherlands

Benno Rensing MD PhD FESC
Department of Cardiology
St Antonius Hospital
Nieuwegein
The Netherlands

MARTIN DUNITZ

© Martin Dunitz Ltd 2002

First published in the United Kingdom in 1997 by
Martin Dunitz Ltd, The Livery House, 7–9 Pratt Street, London NW1 0AE

Tel: +44-(0)20-7482-2202
Fax: +44-(0)20-7267-0159
E-mail: info@dunitz.co.uk
Website: http://www.dunitz.co.uk

Second edition 1998
Reprinted 1998
Third edition 2000
Reprinted 2000

A CIP catalogue record for this book is available from the British Library

ISBN 1-84184-093-9

Distributed in the USA by
Fulfilment Center
Taylor & Francis
7625 Empire Drive
Florence, KY 41042, USA
Toll Free Tel: 1-800-634-7064
Email: cserve@routledge_ny.com

Distributed in Canada by
Taylor & Francis
74 Rolark Drive
Scarborough
Ontario M1R 4G2, Canada
Toll Free Tel: 1-877-226-2237
Email: tal_fran@istar.ca

Distributed in the rest of the world by
ITPS Limited
Cheriton House
North Way, Andover
Hampshire SP10 5BE, UK
Tel: +44-(0)1264 332424
Email: reception@itps.co.uk

Composition by Scribe Design, Gillingham, Kent, UK
Printed and bound in Italy by Printer Trento

CONTENTS

CONTRIBUTORS

Yaron Almagor MD
Director, Cardiac Catheter Unit
Shaare Zedek Medical Center
Department of Cardiology
Jerusalem, Israel

Holger Anhalt
Medical Affairs Manager
Phytis Medical Devices
Berlin, Germany

Tomás Berrazueta
Sales and Marketing Manager
Bolton Medical Inc.
Fair Lawn, NJ, USA

Amadeu Betriu
Professor of Medicine and
Head, Department of Cardiology
Hospital Clinic of Barcelona, University
of Medicine
Barcelona, Spain

Rafael Beyar MD DSC
Dean, Bruce Rappaport Faculty of
Medicine
Director, Division of Invasive
Cardiology, Rambam Medical Center
Dr Phillip and Sarah Gottlieb Chair and
Professor
Technion, Israel Institute of Technology
Haifa, Israel

Peter Boekstegers MD
Hospital Grosshadern, Ludwig-
Maximilians-University,
Medical Clinic I, Munich, Germany

Hans Bonnier MD PhD
Interventional Cardiologist
Department of Interventional Cardiology
Catharina Hospital
Eindhoven, The Netherlands

Andrew J Carter DO
Assistant Professor of Medicine
Interventional Cardiology
Stanford University Medical Center
Stanford, CA, USA

Antonio Colombo MD
Director of Cardiac Catheterization
Laboratory
EMO Centro Cuore Columbus and
Director, Cardiac Catheterization
Laboratory and Interventional
Cardiology, San Raffaele Hospital, Milan
Italy and
Director of Investigational Angioplasty
Lenox Hill Hospital, New York, USA

Marco A Costa MD PhD
Cardiologist, Department of
Interventional Cardiology
Institute Dante Pazzanese of Cardiology
Sao Paolo, Brazil

David C Cumberland FRCR FRCP FRCS
FACC FESC
Consultant Cardiovascular Interventionist
Ampang Puteri Specialist Hospital
Kuala Lumpur, Malaysia

H Richard Davis MSc
Director, Clinical Affairs and Advanced
Research
Orbus Medical Technologies
Hoevelaken, The Netherlands

Lluis Duocastella
Professor of Chemistry and
Managing Technical Director
Iberhospitex SA, Barcelona, Spain

Franz R Eberli MD
Director of Invasive Cardiology
Swiss Cardiovascular Center Bern
University Hospital, Bern, Switzerland

Robert Falotico PhD
Cordis, Johnson and Johnson, Inc.
Warren, NJ, USA

Gennady Fedosenko
University of Wuppertal
Institute of Plasmatechnology
Wuppertal, Germany

David R Fischell PhD
President, Fischell Biomedical LLC,
Fair Haven, NJ, USA

Robert E Fischell ScD
President, IsoStent Inc, Dayton, MD,
USA

Tim A Fischell MD FACC
Director of Cardiovascular Research
Heart Institute at Borgess
Professor of Medicine
Michigan State University
Richland, MI, USA

Peter J Fitzgerald MD PhD
Associate Professor of Medicine
Stanford University Medical Center
Stanford, CA, USA

David P Foley MB MRCPI
Department of Interventional Cardiology
Erasmus University
Heart Center
University Hospital Dijkzigt
Rotterdam
The Netherlands

**Lutz Freiwald Dipl.-Ing Medical
Technique**
General Marketing Manager
Devon Medical
Hamburg, Germany

Eulogio Garcia MD
Director, Department of Interventional
Cardiology
Gregorio Maranon Hospital
Madrid, Spain

Anthony H Gershlick BSC MRCP
Consultant Cardiologist and Honorary
Senior Lecturer
University Hospitals, Leicester, UK

Wim J van der Giessen MD PhD
Erasmus Medical Center Rotterdam,
Department of Cardiology
Thoraxcenter
Rotterdam, the Netherlands

Thomas Glandorf
Polymer Research and Production
Manager
Phytis Medical Devices
Berlin, Germany

Eberhard Grube MD FACC FACA FSCAI
Professor of Medicine and
Chief, Department of
Cardiology/Angiology
Heart Center Siegberg, Germany and
Consulting Professor
Division of Cardiovascular Medicine
Stanford University of Medicine
Stanford, CA, USA

Jürgen Hoge
Administration and Production Director
Phytis Medical Devices
Berlin, Germany

Ronald AM Horvers
President, Blue Medical Devices
Helmond, The Netherlands

Thomas A Ischinger MD FESC FACC
Professor of Medicine
Klinikum München-Bogenhausen
Munich, Germany

Norman T Kanesaka
Engineer and Development Manager
Bolton Medical Inc.
Fair Lawn, NJ, USA

Jacques Koolen MD PhD
Interventional Cardiologist
Department of Interventional Cardiology
Catharina Hospital
Eindhoven, The Netherlands

Guy Leclerc MD
Associate Professor of Research
University of Montreal School of
Medicine and
Director, Cardiac Catheterization
Laboratories
Centre Hospitalier de l'Université de
Montréal
Montréal, PQ, Canada

Jean-Marie Lefebvre MD
Interventional Cardiologist
Clinique de la Louviere
Lille, France

Martin B Leon MD
Chief Executive Officer and President
Cardiovascular Research Foundation
Lenox Hill Hospital
New York, NY, USA

Andrew L Lewis PhD CChem MRSC
Research and Technology Director
Drug Delivery Division
Biocompatibles, Farnham, Surrey, UK

Jurgen Ligthart
Department of Interventional Cardiology
Erasmus University
Heart Center
University Hospital Dijkzigt
Rotterdam
The Netherlands

Ancieto López
President, Iberhospitex SA
Barcelona, Spain

Nico Margaris MD
Department of Interventional Cardiology
Evangelismos Hospital
Athens, Greece

Carlo Di Mario MD PhD FESC FACC
Research and Associate Clinical Director
Interventional Cardiology
San Raffaele Hospital
Milan, Italy

Henk JM Meens
Vice President, Sales and Marketing
Blue Medical Devices
Helmond, The Netherlands

Masakiyo Nobuyoshi MD FACC
Vice Medical Director
Kokura Memorial Hospital, Japan

Michael Orlowski
Master of Biology Bioengineering
Clinical Research
EuroCor
Bonn, Germany

John Ormiston MBChB
Interventional Cardiologist
Mercy and Greenlane Hospitals
Auckland, New Zealand

Isabel Pérez
Biologist and Head of Cardiovascular
Research
and Marketing, Iberhospitex SA
Barcelona
Spain

Brendon J Pittman BA MBA
Product Manager
Boston Scientific
Minneapolis, Minnesota
USA

Nicolaus Reifart MD
JOMED AB
Helsingborg, Sweden

Kobi Richter PhD
Chairman, Medinol Ltd
Tel Aviv
Israel

Philippe Rossi MD
Centre Hospitalier Privé de Clairval
Marseille, France

Martin T Rothman FRCP FACC FESC
Professor of Interventional Cardiology
Director of Cardiac Research and
Development
Cardiac Department
The London Chest Hospital
Barts and the London NHS Trust
London, UK

Anastasios Salachas MD
Department of Interventional Cardiology
Evangelismos
Athens, Greece

Norbert Sass
President & CEO
Phytis AG
Schaffhausen, Switzerland

Marcel Schaefer PhD
Director, Clinical Affairs
Biotronik AG
Bülach, Switzerland

Ivan De Scheerder MD PhD
Professor of Interventional Cardiology
University Hospitals Leuven
Leuven, Belgium

Patrick W Serruys MD PhD FACC FESC
Professor of Interventional Cardiology
Erasmus University
Head, Department of Interventional
Cardiology
Heart Centre
University Hospital Rotterdam-Dijkzigt
Rotterdam, The Netherlands

Ulrich Sigwart MD FRCP FACC FESC
Professor of Medicine
Royal Brompton Hospital
London, UK

Sigmund Silber MD FACC
Professor of Medicine
Dr Müller Hospital, Munich, Germany

J Eduardo Sousa MD PhD
Director, Institute Dante Pazzanese of
Cardiology
Sao Paolo, Brazil

Annette Summers
Director of Business Market and
Development and Sales
Advanced Stent Technologies, Inc.
Pleasanton, CA, USA

Takuro Takagi MD
Research Fellow
EMO Centro Cuore Columbus
Milan, Italy

Hideo Tamai MD
Director, Cardiology Department
Shiga Medical Center for Adults
Moriyama, Shiga, Japan

Israel Tamari MD
Head, Interventional Cardiology
The Heart Institute, Wolfson Medical
Center
Tel Aviv, Israel

Takafumi Tsuji MD
Cardiology Department
Shiga Medical Center for Adults
Moriyama, Shiga, Japan

Susan Veldhof RN
Adrianalaan 171
3053 MB Rotterdam
The Netherlands

Danny de Vries
Senior Product Manager
Occam International B.V.
Eindhoven, The Netherlands

Nigel Wheeldon MBChB MD FRCP FESC
Consultant Cardiologist
South Yorkshire Cardiothoracic Unit
Sheffield, UK and
Visiting Professor of Interventional
Cardiology
Dalian Medical University, Dalian
PR China

Stephan Windecker MD
Attending in Invasive Cardiology
Swiss Cardiovascular Center Bern
University Hospital Bern
Switzerland

1. THE AMG ARTHOS AND ARTHOS^{Inert} CORONARY STENT IMPLANTATION SYSTEMS

amg GmbH, Raesfeld-Erle, Germany

Peter Boekstegers

Description

The coronary stent implantation systems, ARTHOS and ARTHOS^{Inert}, enable easier positioning of the stent during interventions. The stainless steel MAC^{plus} slotted tube stent with its improved design promises to keep restenosis rates low.

The new coronary implantation system ARTHOS^{Inert} offers a stent system with an 'inert' surface, which specifically addresses the problems of nickel, chromium and molybdenum elution. The special refinement process used produces a stent surface, which blocks ion diffusion from the stainless steel. The combination of the ART balloon catheter with the MAC^{plus}-Inert stent in ARTHOS^{Inert} produces a coronary stent implantation system with optimal features for fast and problem-free direct stenting.

History

- 1998 OMEGA stent, MAC stent and their implantation systems are CE marked
- 1999 MAC Carbon stent and coronary implanation system are CE marked
- 2001 MAC^{plus}, MAC^{plus}Inert and the implantation system ARTHOS and ARTHOS^{Inert} are CE marked

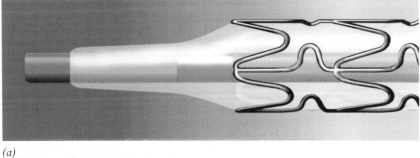

(a)

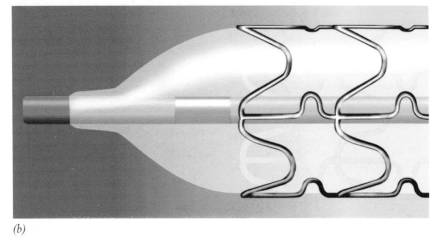

(b)

Figure 1.1: *(a) An absolutely uniform expansion at the beginning of dilatation. (b) At full expansion: soft-end technology and uniform, smooth descending balloon shoulders prevent damage to the healthy intima.*

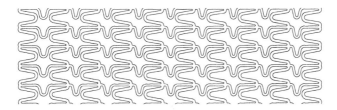

Figure 1.2: *Design of the MAC^plus small stent.*

ARTHOS stent technical specifications

Material composition:	Stainless steel
Degree of radiopacity:	Moderate
Ferromagnetism:	Non-ferromagnetic (MRI safe)
MRI:	Should not be examined by MRI for the first 3 months after implantation
Metallic surface area expanded:	Small: 10.9–19.6% Large: 12.8–23.0%
Stent design:	Laser-cut slotted tube
Strut design:	Connected loops
Strut dimensions:	125 μm
Profiles on the balloon:	1.06 mm (average)
Longitudinal flexibility:	Excellent
Percentage shortening on expansion:	1.6% small 1.3% large
Expansion range:	2.5 to 5.0 mm
Degree of recoil:	1.84% small 1.86% large
Radial strength:	High
Currently available diameters:	2.5 to 5.0 mm
Currently available lengths:	10, 14, 18, 24, 28 mm
Currently available sizes:	Small (2.5–3.0 mm) Large (3.5–4.0 mm)
Recrossability of implanted stent	Good

3

ARTHOS^{Inert} stent technical specifications

Material composition:	Stainless steel with 'inert' surface
Degree of radiopacity:	Moderate
Ferromagnetism:	Non-ferromagnetic (MRI safe)
MRI:	Should not be examined by MRI for the first 3 months after implantation
Metallic surface area expanded:	Small: 10.9–19.6% Large: 12.8–23.0%
Stent design:	Laser-cut slotted tube
Strut design:	Connected loops
Strut dimensions:	125 μm
Profiles on the balloon:	1.06 mm (average)
Longitudinal flexibility:	Excellent
Percentage shortening on expansion:	1.6% small 1.3% large
Expansion range:	2.5 to 5.0 mm
Degree of recoil:	1.84% small 1.86% large
Radial strength:	High
Currently available diameters:	2.5 to 5.0 mm
Currently available lengths:	10, 14, 18, 24, 28 mm
Currently available sizes:	Small (2.5–3.0 mm) Large (3.5–4.0 mm)
Recrossability of implanted stent	Good

Indications for use

- Direct stenting of de novo lesions
- Restenosis
- Bifurcation stenoses
- Sub-optimal PTCA results
- Failed PTCA (e.g. with acute occlusion)

The advantages of the MAC*plus*:

- High flexibility
- Top quality inner/outer surface finish
- High radial strength
- No significant shortening
- Low crimping profile

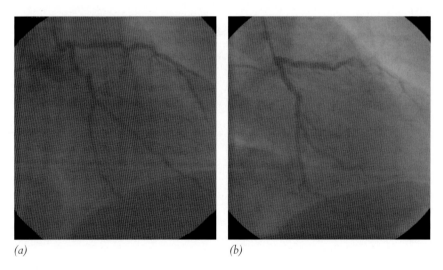

(a)   (b)

Figure 1.3:
(a) High grade eccentric stenosis in the CX with 90° descent from main branch.
(b) Direct stenting with ARTHOS delivery system.

Clinical development from MAC to MAC^{plus}

In an initial evaluation 74 MAC stents were implanted into 70 patients.[1] Stents were available in 9, 17, 27 and 36 mm lengths. Control angiography was performed after 6 months.

Lesion characterization (according to AHA): 1x Type A, 2x Type B1, 44x Type B2, 23x Type C. Stenosis localization: 1x LM, 26x LAD, 18x RCX, 24x RCA; 33x proximal, 32x central, 5x distal.

Average degree of stenosis 88.8 per cent, average reference vessel diameter 3.09 mm, average length of stenosis 13.2 mm.

All 74 stents could be deployed (100 per cent); stent expansion took place at 3–4 bar , average implantation pressure was 12.3 bar (10–14 atm), all stents could be expanded without visible recoil, no acute complications.

6 months follow up:

Diameter of stenosis	50–75%	75–99%	100%	Total restenosis (> 50%)	Re-PTCA	CAGB
Number of patients	2	9	1	12	10	0
Restenosis rate	2.9	12.9	1.4	17.1	14.2	0

Between March 1999 and June 1999, 143 patients were treated by implantation of MAC stents in 24 centers;[2] 6 month follow-up data was obtained in 130 patients with 137 lesions. MAC stents (2.5–4.0 mm diameter, 9–36 mm length) were pre-mounted on a rapid exchange delivery system. One stent was implanted per lesion.

Stent implantation was immediately successful in all 137 lesions (diameter stenosis < 50%). Procedure-related complications including death, acute myocardial infarction, and TLR did not occur.

Indications for coronary stenting were: elective in 93 lesions (67.9%), sub-optimal result after balloon angioplasty in 35 lesions (25.5%), acute and subacute closures in nine lesions (6.9%): de novo in 132 lesions (96.4%) and restenotic lesions in five cases (3.6%). Lesion types (ACC/AHA) were: type A 25 (18.2%), type B1 37(27.0%), type B2 56 (40.9%) and type C 19 (13.9%). Lesion length was 13.6 ± 6.2 mm and vessel diameter 3.2 ± 0.4 mm. Pre-procedure, minimal lumen diameter was 0.6 ± 0.3 mm. MLD post implantation was 3.2 ± 0.4 mm.

Major cardiac events during 6–month follow-up period were: one death, one acute myocardial infarction, 13 (10%) clinically documented cases of recurrent ischemia. Follow-up coronary angiography was performed for 112 lesions in 110 patients (84.6%). Minimal lumen diameter was 2.1 ± 0.8 mm with stenosis diameter of 32 ± 24%. Restenosis (> 50% diameter stenosis) occurred in 21 lesions of 20 patients (18.2%) and TLR (8x balloon angioplasty and 2x stent implantation) was performed in 10 patients (7.7%).

In a further pilot study[3] 70 stainless steel stents were implanted, of which 20 stents had an *'Inert'* surface. The stents were available in the sizes 3.0 and 3.5 × 16 mm, the stent carrier system used was identical. The degree of stenosis was determined with on-line QCA, and procedural data documented. Vessels affected (mostly LAD) and lesion characteristics in both groups were similar with mostly type B2 and type C lesions. Angiographic control was repeated after 6 months.

19/20 *'Inert'* stents and 48/50 'plain' stents could be successfully implanted. There were no acute complications.

6 months follow up:

	Patient number	Stenosis diameter				Restenosis rate
		0–50%	50–75%	75–99%	100%	(%)
Stent with 'inert' surface	19	100	0	0	0	0
Stent without 'inert' surface	48	83.3	2.1	12.5	2.1	16.70

References

1. Voigt BJ, Pfitzner P, Boeck U *et al*. The MAC stent: first experiences and results. *German J Cardiol* 2000;**89**(suppl 6).

2. Takh S-J. Korea – a multicenter trial: six-month clinical and angiographic follow-up results of MAC stent study. Accepted for publication in *The Korean Circulation Journal*.

3. Voigt BJ, Paul M, Pfitzner P *et al*. Does an *'inert'* surface affect the restenosis rate of stainless steel stents? A pilot study.

2. THE ANTARES STARFLEX® CORONARY STENT SYSTEM

InFlow Dynamics AG, Munich, Germany

Carlo di Mario

Description	Starflex design is homogeneous, multicellular stent structure with alternating stiff and flex segments for excellent longitudinal flexibility.

History	• 1999 launch of Antares Coronary with Flex-Plus design • 2000 modification of Flex-Plus design to Starflex design • September 2000 CE-mark and launch of Antares Starflex in Germany and internationally • End of 2000 first human implants in approximately 2000 patients • Beginning of 2001 launch of Antares Starflex Profile (Starflex design with 2-step-shoulder balloon) • 2001 Worldwide market penetration

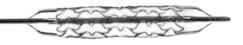

Figure 2.1: *Expanded Antares Starflex® coronary stent delivery system.*

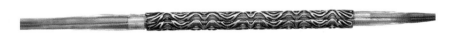

Figure 2.2: *Crimped Antares Starflex® coronary stent delivery system.*

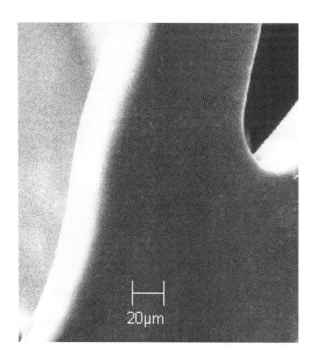

Figure 2.3: *Electron microscopy of Antares Starflex® stent.*

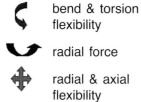

ⵦ bend & torsion flexibility

radial force

radial & axial flexibility

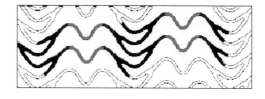

Figure 2.4: *Schematic drawing of Antares Starflex® stent design showing the alternating stiff and flex elements which combine flexibility and radial force.*

Technical specifications

Material composition:	316 L stainless steel, surface polished
Degree of radiopacity (grade):	Medium
Ferromagnetism:	Non-ferromagnetic
MRI:	MRI-proof
Metallic surface area:	Dependent on expanded diameter (13–17%)
Stent design:	Homogeneous, multicellular stent structure, 'Starflex'-design
Strut design:	Oval strut cross-section
Strut dimensions:	90 × 85 µm
Strut angles:	Dependent on diameter
Strut thickness:	90 µm
Crossing profile(s) on the balloons:	2.5 mm balloon diameter: 0.0382 inch 4.0 mm balloon diameter: 0.0471 inch
Longitudinal flexibility:	Excellent
Percentage shortening (on delivery):	0%
Percentage shortening on expansion:	< 3%
Expansion range:	2.5–4.5 mm
Degree of recoil (shape memory):	< 3%
Radial force:	High
Currently available diameters:	2.5–4.0 mm
Currently available lengths mounted/implanted:	8 mm, 12 mm, 16 mm, 20 mm, 24 mm, 32 mm
Currently available sizes: balloon diameter	Each length for 2.5/3.0/3.5/4.0 mm
Recrossability of implanted stent:	Excellent
Other non-coronary types available:	Peripheral stents: Antares Endovascular OTW Antares Renal RX

Tips and tricks for delivery

The low profile of the stent allows easy delivery through 6 French and large lumen 5 French guiding catheters. Before expansion the stent is clearly visible on the delivery balloon while visibility after expansion is dependent on the patient's characteristics and quality of the X-ray system. The stent delivery system is suitable for direct stenting, but extremely tortuous vessels and calcification should be avoided. The balloon is a high pressure semi-compliant balloon easily expandable up to 14–16 atmospheres. If oversized balloons are used, slight withdrawal of the balloon is recommended as a minimal dog-bone effect can be present in highly resistant lesions. The absence of specific techniques of crimping is an advantage as the balloon will easily become free from the stent after deployment and can be used for postdilatation or dilatation elsewhere in the vessel.

Indications for use

- In patients eligible for balloon angioplasty with symptomatic ischemic heart disease characterized by discrete de novo and restenosed coronary artery lesions with reference vessel diameter from 2.5 mm to 4.5 mm.
- In elective implantation and in treatment of acute or threatened closure associated with a coronary intervention, including saphenous vein graft.

Why I like my stent

The stent is the product of careful design from a selected group of engineers and expert reviews from practising physicians: it is a classical slotted tubular stent with a design optimized to allow good scaffolding and maintain side-branch access. The stent has sufficient radial strength and wall coverage to deliver a smooth vessel contour also in unstable plaques with soft irregular contours. It has a flexibility that is comparable to other well-known slotted tube stents.

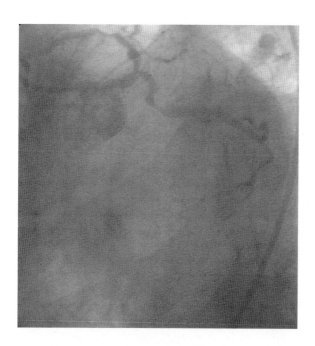

Figure 2.5:
Eccentric lesion in a
very tortuous proximal
left circumflex artery.

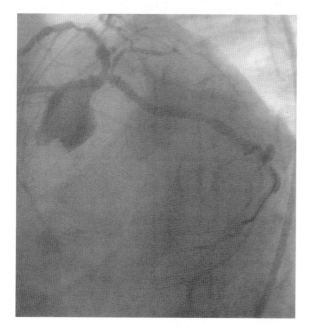

Figure 2.6:
Circumflex coronary
artery after treatment
with a 16 mm 3.5 mm
Antares Starflex® stent.

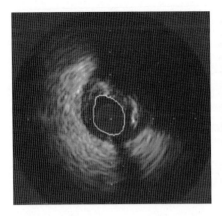 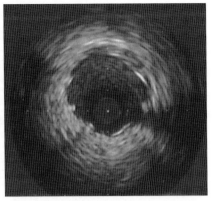

Figure 2.7: *IVUS image before stenting of the circumflex lesion.*

Figure 2.8: *IVUS image of a fully deployed Antares Starflex® stent.*

Ongoing clinical trials

- MOONLIGHT study: European prospective, multi-centre registry of 120 consecutive patients with single or multi-vessel disease. Follow-up 1 and 6 months. Start: March 2001.
- Clinical evaluation of Lunar Coronary Stent System at Swiss Cardiovascular Center Bern, Switzerland.
- Clinical evaluation of Lunar Coronary Stent System in Argentina and Brazil with 40 patients.

3. THE AST SLK-VIEW STENT AND DELIVERY SYSTEM

Advanced Stent Technologies, Pleasanton, CA, USA

Annette Summers

Definition	The SLK-View stent is indicated for improving coronary luminal diameter while maintaining side aperture access in patients with symptomatic ischemic disease due to discrete *de novo* lesions in native coronary arteries involving a major side branch (length < 17 mm & side branch diameter > 2 mm) with a reference vessel diameter of 3.0 to 3.75 mm. The stent is a 316L stainless steel flexible slotted tube stent with a side aperture located between the proximal and distal section. The purpose of the aperture is to allow access to the side branch vessel after deployment. The stent is pre-mounted and is expanded with balloon inflation.

History	• July 29, 1998 First in vivo experience with swine • March 6, 2000 Venezuelan and Korean clinical studies initiated • May 16, 2001 GLP study in swine coronary arteries initiated

Indications for use

The SLK-View stent is indicated for improving coronary luminal diameter while maintaining side aperture access in patients with symptomatic ischemic disease due to discrete *de novo* lesions in native coronary arteries involving a major side branch (length < 17 mm & side branch diameter > 2 mm) with a reference vessel diameter of 3.0 to 3.75 mm.

AST SLK-View stent technical specifications

Material composition:	316L stainless steel
Degree of radiopacity (grade):	Moderate
Ferromagnetism:	Yes
MRI:	N/A
Metallic surface area unexpanded:	expanded: 13–14%
Metallic cross-sectional area:	0.000071–0.000573 sq. inch
Stent design:	Serpentine w/Expandable Side Hole
Strut design:	'C' and 'S'
Strut dimensions:	0.002–0.004 inch
Strut thickness:	0.0045 inch
Profile(s): non-expanded (uncrimped): expanded: on the balloons:	0.061 inch 3.0–3.3 mm, 3.5–3.8 mm 0.055 inch
Longitudinal flexibility:	Moderate
Percentage shortening on expansion:	< 10%
Expansion range:	3.0–3.3 mm, 3.5–3.8 mm
Degree of recoil (shape memory):	< 5%
Radial force:	Moderate
Currently available diameters:	3.0 mm, 3.5 mm
Currently available lengths mounted/implanted: unmounted:	17 mm, 18 mm
Currently available sizes:	3.0 mm × 20 mm, 3.5 mm × 20 mm
Recrossability of implanted stent:	Moderate

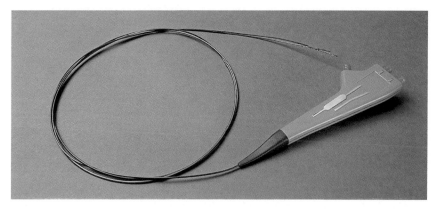

Figure 3.1: Delivery system.

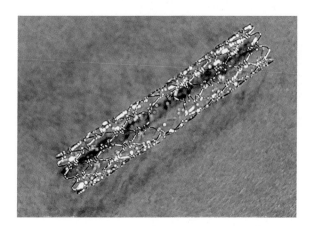

Figure 3.2: Expanded stent.

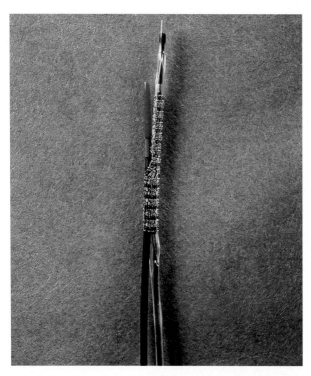

Figure 3.3:
SLK-View stent.

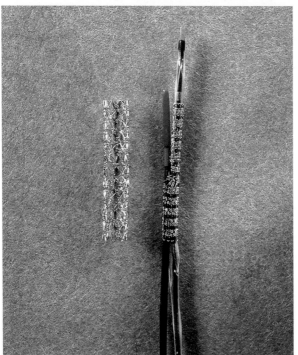

Figure 3.4:
SLK-View stent.

Why I like my stent

- Maintains side access to a side branch
- Radiopacity makes for easy placement in main branch and allows alignment to the side branch.

Clinical trials

On-going:
- Two single-center registry clinical research studies outside of the US
- Animal Research and Development
- GLP with a control

Planned:
- European Feasibility – 30 patient single center registry
- US IDE Feasibility trial – 30 patient multicenter registry
- US IDE Pivotal trial – 300 patient 3 arm, multicenter, randomization protocol with a control

This SLK-View device is an investigation device and is not FDA approved for sale in the United States.

4. THE BeStent™2 Stent

Medtronic AVE, Santa Rosa, CA, USA

Rafael Beyar and Patrick W Serruys

Definition	A laser-cut balloon expandable, stainless steel stent with solid gold radiopaque end markers. The BeStent2 is mounted on a semi-compliant balloon with Discrete Technology™. Rapid Exchange (outside US only), Rapid Exchange with Perfusion (US only), and Over the Wire (US only) platforms are available.

Description	The stent is characterized by flexible 'S' crowns and longitudinal 'V' crowns that cross each other in a unique junction which undergoes rotation during expansion. This unique expansion mechanism distributes stress and minimizes foreshortening and recoil. The stent has two radiopaque gold markers for visibility of the stent ends, allowing for precise positioning.

History	• 1996 First human implant of BeStent • 1999 BeStent Brava launched • 2000 BeStent2 clinical trial completed with 227 patients • 2000 BeStent2 launched in Europe, Asia, Canada and USA

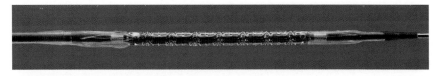

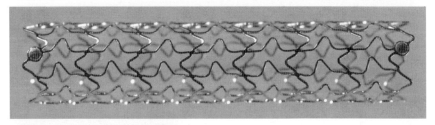

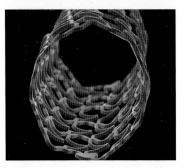

Figure 4.1: *Above: the mounted BeStent2 balloon expandable stent (upper). The unique gold markers are clearly seen at the stent ends. The expanded stent is shown (lower). Left is an SEM showing the scaffolding provided by the BeStent2 architecture.*

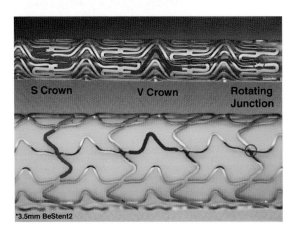

Figure 4.2: *These images show the stent design and the mechanism of stent expansion. As the stent expands, the V crowns and S crowns straighten both in the longitudinal and radial directions. The rotating junction distributes stress and minimizes foreshortening and recoil.*

BeStent2 stent technical specifications

Material composition:	316 L stainless steel
Degree of radiopacity:	Moderate, compensated by radiopaque gold markers at stent ends
Ferromagnetism:	Non-ferromagnetic (MRI safe**)
Vessel wall coverage:	12–17%
Stent design:	A laser-cut tube with no welding points
Strut design:	Rectangular
Strut dimensions:	S crown 0.085 mm thick & 0.95 mm wide. Longitudinal V crown 0.085 mm thick & 0.070 mm wide
Longitudinal flexibility:	High
Percentage shortening on expansion:	~0% (between gold markers)
Expansion range:	2.5 mm* – 4.5 mm
Degree of recoil (shape memory):	≤ 2.2%
Radial force:	Resist at least 550 mmHg
Current available lengths:	9, 12, 15, 18, 24 & 30 mm
Current available sizes:	2.5*, 3.0, 3.5, 4.0 mm
Recrossability of implanted stents:	Excellent

*2.5 mm not available in the USA.

**Magnetic resonance imaging should not be performed until the implanted stent has been completely endothelialized (8 weeks) in order to minimize the risk of stent migration under a strong magnetic field. The stent may cause artifacts in MRI scans due to the distortion of the magnetic field.

BeStent2 rapid exchange delivery system (outside US only)

Mechanism of deployment:	Balloon expandable
Mechanism of expanding:	The unique rotating junction expands the stent uniformly and distributes stress. This also minimizes foreshortening and recoil.
Minimal internal diameter of guiding catheter:	0.058 inch (5F)
Delivery system:	Pre-mounted on a semi-compliant rapid exchange delivery system with Discrete Technology™.
Balloon material:	AVE proprietary balloon material
Guidewire lumen:	0.014 inch (0.36 mm)
Protective sheath:	None
Position of radiopaque markers:	Gold markers are positioned on the stent ends. Balloon markers proximal and distal to the stent.
Rated burst pressure of the balloon:	16 atm
Delivery balloon compliance:	Semi-compliant
Longitudinal flexibility:	High
Recommended deployment pressure:	8 atm
Further dilatation comment:	At physician's discretion

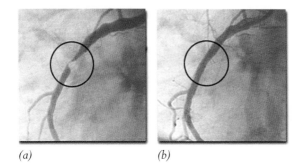 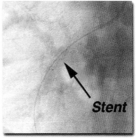

(a)   (b)

Figure 4.3:
(a) Pre-stenting; (b) Post-stenting using BeStent2.

Indications for use

The BeStent2 is indicated for improving coronary luminal diameter in patients with symptomatic ischemic heart disease due to discrete *de novo* lesions (length ≤ 30 mm) in native coronary arteries with reference vessel diameters ranging from 2.5 mm to 4.0 mm.

Why I like the BeStent2

We find this stent extremely friendly, and with a unique angiographic appearance combining excellent scaffolding with end-markers that is not shared by other stents. Navigating tortuous anatomies is possible due to the high flexibility, and the new delivery system that makes stent slippage on the balloon almost impossible. The low profile and the secure mounting of the BeStent2 on the balloon has made crossing tight lesions easier. The end-markers allow precise placement, especially in situations in which this is critical, like side-branches and bifurcations. The angiographic image post procedure shows a homogeneous expanded stent with an even scaffolding of the vessel wall without compromising on side-branch access. One can easily stent over angled segments without the fear for plaque prolapse, which may happen with different stent designs. Solutions for the daily challenges in the cath lab are incorporated in the design of the BeStent2 and make it a highly versatile stent for the treatment of the widest range of lesions.

Completed and ongoing clinical studies with the BeStent/BeStent2

Acronym/author	Design	Patients	Status/results
BEST[1]	Randomized vs. Palmaz Schatz stent	325	Single de novo lesions. BeStent: RR 16.5%, TLR @ 6 m 4.1%
Rose[2]	Registry	120	Single de novo lesions. Mean vessel diameter 2.85 ± 0.52 mm, RR 21.5%, TLR @ 6 m 10.0%
Roguin et al[3]	Registry	100	Relatively complex lesions. EFS @ 12 m 82%
Gruberg et al[4]	Registry	40	Open criteria. No. events @ 30 days.
Baldus et al[5]	Registry	117	Complex lesions. Successful stent deployment 94%
BESMART[6]	Small vessels Randomized vs. balloon	381	RR @ 6 m: stent 22.7%; balloon 48.8% ($p = 0.0001$) TLR @ 6 m: stent 13%; balloon 25% ($p = 0.016$)
SISA[7]	Small vessels Randomized vs. balloon	352	MACE @ discharge: stent 3.0%; balloon 7.1% ($p = 0.076$) MACE @ 6 m: stent 18.3%; balloon 22.0% ($p =$ ns) RR @ 6 m: stent 28.0%; balloon 32.9% ($p =$ ns)
RAP[8]	Small vessels Randomized vs. balloon	426	RR @ 6 m: stent 27%; balloon 37% TLR @ 6 m: stent 12.2%; balloon 22.3% EFS @ 6 m: stent 86.4%; balloon 74.9%
SISCA[9]	Small vessels Randomized vs. balloon	145	EFS @ 30 days: 98.6% for both groups EFS @ 6 m: stent 90.5%; balloon 76.1% ($p = 0.025$)
BeStent2 trial[10]	Registry	227	Lesion length max. 28 mm. Procedure success 97.8% MACE @ 30 days: 3.6% MACE @ 180 days: 12.1%
Convertible	Randomized	200	Ongoing. Predilatation versus direct stenting

TLR, Target lesion revascularization; RR, Restenosis rate; MACE, Major adverse coronary events; EFS, Event-free survival

References

1. BEST-Study. Data provided by manufacturer.

2. Suryapranata H, Boland JL, Pieper M *et al.* Clinical and angiographic results with the BeStent. The Registry for Optimal BeStent Evaluation (ROSE) Trial. *Int J Cardiovasc Intervent* 2000;**3**:21–8.

3. Roguin A, Gruberg L, Markiewicz W *et al.* One-year clinical follow-up with the serpentine balloon expandable stent: report of the first 100 patients. *Coron Artery Dis* 1999;**10**:421–5.

4. Gruberg L, Grenadier E, Miller H *et al.* First clinical experience with the premounted balloon-expandable serpentine stent: acute angiographic and intermediate-term clinical results. *Catheter Cardiovasc Interv* 1999;**46**:249–53.

5. Baldus S, Hamm CW, Köster R *et al.* Initial single-center experience with a new intracoronary stent. *Int J Cardiovasc Intervent* 1998;**1**:99–104.

6. Koning RA. In-hospital results and six-months clinical and angiographic follow-up of coronary stenting in small coronary arteries: final results of the BeStent in small arteries (BESMART) study. *J Am Coll Cardiol* 2000;**36**:314–15 (abstract).

7. Doucet S, Schalij MJ, Vrolix MCM *et al.* Stent placement to prevent restenosis after angioplasty in small coronary arteries. For the Stent In Small Arteries (SISA) trial investigators. *Circulation* 2000;102–663 (abstract).

8. Restenosis en Arteries Pequeñas Study. E. Garcia TCT 2000.

9. Stenting in small coronary artery study (SISCA). Data provided by R. Moer.

10. BeStent2 Revascularization Trial (Heart Knows No Borders program). Data provided by manufacturer.

5. THE B*IODIVYSIO*® AS, OC AND SV STENT RANGE WITH PC TECHNOLOGY™

Biocompatibles Ltd, Farnham, Surrey, UK

David C Cumberland and Ulrich Sigwart

Description	Balloon expandable, laser sculpted from stainless steel tubes, comprising an interlocking arrowhead design. Three derivations of the design — Added Support (AS), Open Cell (OC), and Small Vessel (SV). All stents are coated with phosphorylcholine (PC) Technology with or without local drug delivery capability.

History	The Bio*div*Ysio range of stents with PC Technology was developed by DivYsio Solutions Ltd in conjunction with Biocompatibles Ltd. The stents are coated with Biocompatibles' proprietary coating, PC Technology, which has local drug delivery capability.

	• September 1996	First human coronary implant of Bio*div*Ysio
	• December 1997	European CE mark approval of Bio*div*Ysio
	• August 1998	Premounted Bio*div*Ysio launched
	• August 1999	Bio*div*Ysio SV launched
	• November 1999	Bio*div*Ysio with drug delivery capability received CE mark approval
	• September 2000	FDA approval for 15 mm Bio*div*Ysio AS
	• November 2000	Bio*div*Ysio Matrix LO and Matrix HI with specific molecular weight drug delivery received CE mark approval
	• March 2001	New delivery system for Bio*div*Ysio SV with enhanced push and track
	• June 2001	New delivery system for Bio*div*Ysio AS and OC with enhanced push and track

Indications for use

Indications are currently as for other coronary stents. Preclinical and clinical studies suggest that PC Technology may confer added clinical advantage in terms of thrombo-resistance, safety and long-term biocompatibility. Additional elastic and friction studies demonstrate that PC coating is highly durable and stable. These results suggest a particular role in adverse or high risk subsets. At present there are three stent designs available:

1) Added Support design (Bio*divYsio* AS), which has a longitudinal member within the open space of each arrowhead (refer to attached pictures of stents) to confer greater support,

2) Open Cell design (Bio*divYsio* OC), which has greater flexibility and potential for side branch access (refer to attached pictures of stents), and

3) Small Vessel design (Bio*divYsio* SV) which mimics the Open Cell design in terms of structure, but is made from a 1.0 mm stainless steel tube, as opposed to a 1.6 mm stainless steel tube for the other two designs, which affords a tailored fit within small coronaries (< 2.75 mm in diameter). The results of the 2 mm diameter stent registry are awaited.

There are six elements circumferentially, for use in vessels between 2.0 and 4.25 mm in diameter. All three stent designs are coated with PC Technology, which is available with or without local drug delivery capability.

Why I like my stent

- Good balance between flexibility and vessel support.
- Ability for low pressure, symmetrical deployment.
- Cosmetically attractive appearances on angiography and intravascular ultrasound.
- Side-branch encroachment is particularly straightforward with the Bio*divYsio*; if needed, access to side branches is relatively easy.
- Ready ability to re-cross the implanted stent with a second delivery system.
- Future family of stents based on fundamental design.
- Local drug delivery capabilities, through Biocompatibles' proprietary coating, have the ability to encompass the many processes associated with restenosis: injury, migration, proliferation and healing.

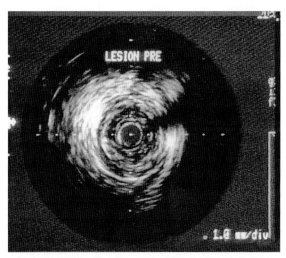

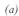
(a)

Figure 5.1: *IVUS images of lesion in saphenous vein graft. (a) before; (b) after stenting. The even, circular appearance on IVUS is characteristic of this stent.*

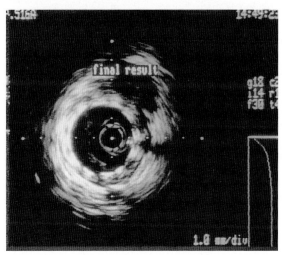
(b)

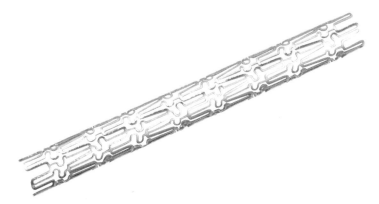

Figure 5.2: Added support (BiodivYsio AS).

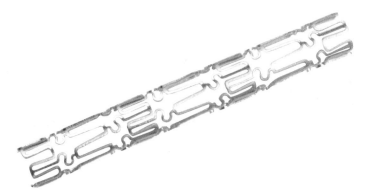

Figure 5.3: Open cell (BiodivYsio OC).

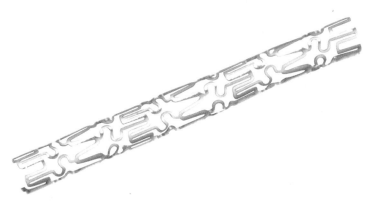

Figure 5.4: Small vessel (BiodivYsio SV).

Clinical trials

Global Stent Registry: Worldwide open registry of implantation with no inclusion or exclusion criteria, i.e., 'real world' stenting. 229 stents in 187 patients in 17 centres. Clinical follow-up. Major adverse cardiac events (MACE at 30 days: 7.1%, target lesion for revascularization (TLR) at 6 months, 6.4%).

Safety and Performance Study: 150 patients, 8 European centres. Single lesion suitable for 15 mm or 28 mm stent. Clinical follow-up. Results at 6 months: MACE 8%, TVR 6%.

SOPHOS Study: 425 patients, 24 centres in Europe, Canada and South America. Single lesions, suitable for 15 mm stent, similar to those in 'BENESTENT I' trial. The first 200 patients (SOPHOS A) have had angiographic and clinical follow-up; the later cohort (SOPHOS B) just clinical assessment. Results: SOPHOS A: overall restenosis 17.7%; in the first quartile of vessel sizes (1.3–2.6 mm diameter) restenosis 20%. SOPHOS A+B MACE 13% at 6 months.

SPEEDS: Canadian Safety and Effectiveness Study. Native vessels 2.5 mm to 4.0 mm and lesions up to 23 mm long. 437 patients. 6-month clinical follow up. Interim composite endpoint: MACE 9.7%. Sub-Acute Stent Thrombosis 0.5%.

DISTINCT (US IDE): 35 centres in USA and Canada. Randomized prospective study of the BiodivYsio stent and Multi-Link Duet®. 622 patients. Single de novo lesions up to 25 mm long. 6 month angiographic follow-up. Binary restenosis: BiodivYsio arm: 19.9%; Multi-Link 20.13% (p value – no significance). Subacute thrombosis (SAT ($\leq$ 30 days): BiodivYsio arm: 0%, Multi-Link Duet arm: 0.65% (p value – No Significance).

Small Vessel Registry: 150 lesions (143 patients). 19 centres. Prospective, single-arm registry of the BiodivYsio SV stent. Single de novo lesions up to 15 mm in length and 2.0 to 2.75 mm diameter. 30-day clinical follow up and 6-month clinical and angiographic follow-up.

Multi-Link Duet is the trademark of Guidant Inc.

The Bio*divY*sio AS (added support) stent technical specifications

Material composition:	316 L stainless steel coated with phosphorylcholine (PC Technology™)
Degree of radiopacity (grade):	Moderate
Ferromagnetism:	Non-ferromagnetic (MRI safe)
Metallic surface area (metal: artery expanded):	@ 3.0 mm = 18% @ 3.5 mm = 16% @ 4.0 mm = 14%
Stent design:	Interlocking arrowheads with rectangular, rounded edge struts
Strut dimensions:	0.002–0.003 inch (0.05–0.08 mm) wide and 0.004 inch (0.09 mm) thick
Profile: non-expanded (uncrimped):	1.6 mm
Longitudinal flexibility:	Moderate
Percentage shortening on expansion:	< 4% (1% @ 3 mm diameter)
Expansion range:	2.75 to 4.25 mm
Degree of recoil (shape memory):	1% at 4.0 mm diameter
Radial force (to collapse):	High (> 1.5 N)
Currently available diameters:	2.75, 3.0, 3.5 and 4.0 mm
Currently available lengths:	8, 11 and 15 mm

The Bio*divY*sio OC (open cell) stent technical specifications

Material composition:	316 L stainless steel coated with phosphorylcholine (PC Technology™)
Degree of radiopacity (grade):	Moderate
Ferromagnetism:	Non-ferromagnetic (MRI safe)
Metallic surface area (metal: artery expanded):	@ 3.0 mm = 12% @ 3.5 mm = 11% @ 4.0 mm = 9%
Stent design:	Interlocking arrowheads with rectangular, rounded edge struts
Strut dimensions:	0.002–0.003 inch (0.05–0.08 mm) wide and 0.004 inch (0.09 mm) thick
Profile: non-expanded (uncrimped):	1.6 mm
Longitudinal flexibility:	High
Percentage shortening on expansion:	< 4% (1% @ 3 mm diameter)
Expansion range:	2.75 to 4.25 mm
Degree of recoil (shape memory):	1% at 4.0 mm diameter
Radial force (to collapse):	High (> 1.5 N)
Currently available diameters:	2.75, 3.0, 3.5 and 4.0 mm
Currently available lengths:	8, 11, 15, 18, 22 and 28 mm

The Bio*div*Ysio SV (small vessel) stent technical specifications

Material composition:	316 L stainless steel coated with phosphorylcholine (PC Technology™)
Degree of radiopacity (grade):	Moderate
Ferromagnetism:	Non-ferromagnetic (MRI safe)
Metallic surface area (metal: artery expanded):	@ 2.0 mm = 15% @ 2.5 mm = 12%
Stent design:	Interlocking arrowheads with rectangular, rounded edge struts
Strut dimensions:	0.001–0.002 inch (0.03–0.05 mm) wide and 0.002 inch (0.06 mm) thick
Profile: non-expanded (uncrimped):	1.0 mm
Longitudinal flexibility:	High
Percentage shortening on expansion:	< 4% (1% @ 2 mm diameter)
Expansion range:	2.0 to 2.75 mm
Degree of recoil (shape memory):	1% at 3.0 mm diameter
Radial force (to collapse):	High (> 1.5 N)
Currently available diameters:	2.0, 2.25 and 2.5 mm
Currently available lengths:	7, 10, 15, and 18 mm

Review of Published Literature on the Bio*div*Ysio stent coated with PC Technology from Biocompatibles

Clinical evaluations with the Bio*div*Ysio stents started in September 1996. The SOPHOS study commenced in April 1997 and investigated the safety and effectiveness of the 15 mm bare stent in a large formal registry of 425 patients.[11] Half the patients (SOPHOS A, $n = 200$), were assigned angiographic follow-up (assessed by off-line QCA) at 6 months, the other group (SOPHOS B, $n = 225$), were clinically assessed. All patients were observed clinically at discharge, 30 days and 9 months. Patient selection was restricted to short (< 12 mm) *de novo* lesions in single vessels (reference vessel diameter 2.98 ± 0.48 mm, lesion length 8.4 ± 2.86 mm). Minimum lumen diameter pre-/post-procedure and at follow-up was 1.0 ± 0.32; 2.69 ± 0.37; 1.91 ± 0.71 mm respectively. The primary endpoint was the incidence of major adverse cardiac events (MACE) at 6 months, which was 13.4%. Secondary endpoints included among others 6 months binary restenosis, which was 17.7% ($n = 181$ matched lesions). The incidence of MACE and binary restenosis is similar to other comparable reference studies.

Bio*divYsio* stents have been evaluated in 'real-world' clinical settings outside the constraints of formal clinical trials.[9,12] Zheng et al studied 224 patients who underwent elective (67%) or bail-out implantation of 303 Bio*divYsio* stents (15 or 28 mm in length) in 286 lesions. Galli et al collated data on 218 patients treated with a total of 258 stents (15 and 28 mm stents) in 233 lesions. In these studies patients were predominantly those from higher risk groups. Zheng et al reported that 62% of patients had unfavourable anatomy (type B2 and C lesions), 50% had thrombus present and/or chronic total occlusion (24.8%).[13] Procedural success was 99.3% ($n = 284$) of lesions treated. The cohort reported by Galli et al comprised 50% of patients with unstable angina and 13% with acute MI. Procedural success was 99.5% of patients ($n = 212$). Zheng et al reported clinical restenosis in 6.1% (8/132) patients, and target vessel revascularization in 5.4% (8/147 lesions). There were two in-hospital deaths (0.9%) and one subacute thrombosis (0.4%). Galli et al reported 87% of patients were asymptomatic at 6 months. There was one death due to subacute thrombosis on day 7 and three MIs were recorded. Both authors concluded that the Bio*divYsio* stent was safe and effective in high risk clinical or anatomical situations.

Kuiper and Nordrehaug (2000) evaluated 50 patients with totally occluded single vessels treated with the Bio*divYsio* stent.[14] Patients were given reverse heparin treatment with protamine sulphate following intervention to improve patient mobility. Overall, 50 patients with stable angina and a single occluded artery (one unprotected left main, 15 LAD, 11 left circumflex, 23 right) were observed. Patients were given 25 mg protamine sulphate, 250 mg of oral ticlopidine. One stent thrombus was detected 30 minutes post-procedure and was treated with a balloon. Another patient underwent CABG for a non-stent related problem. Treatment improved mobility. Maximal exercise capacity increased from 128 ± 42 to 160 ± 45 watts ($p < 0.05$). Heparin reversal with protamine sulphate following treatment of total occlusions with the Bio*divYsio* stent enabled early mobilization of patients. Complication rates were low.

The Bio*divYsio* stent has been evaluated in a randomized clinical trial, DISTINCT (Feit *et al.*, 2001).[15] In this North American study, 622 patients were randomized to either the 15 mm Bio*divYsio* stent ($n = 313$) or the Multi-Link Duet ($n = 309$, 8, 13, 18, 23, 28 mm lengths). Primary objective was determination of equivalence with respect to the composite endpoint of target vessel failure (TVF; comprising death, recurrent MI, clinically driven revascularization) at 6 months. Angiographic criteria selected patients with *de novo* lesion < 25 mm long with reference vessel of > 3.0 – < 4.0 mm (visual), > 2.75–< 4.0 mm (QCA). Reference vessel diameter Bio*div*Ysio was 2.95 ± 0.48 mm, Duet 2.97 ± 0.53 mm. Up to two, 15 mm Bio*div*Ysio stents were permitted whereas Duet stents were limited to appropriately sized single stents. The incidence of TVF for the Bio*div*Ysio 15 mm pre-mounted stent was 8.3% (25/312) and for the Duet was 7.4% (23/309). Angiographic follow-up was assigned to 200 patients per arm. Binary restenosis was 19.9% (29/146) for the Bio*div*Ysio and 20.1% (30/149) for the Duet ($p = $ NS). MACE free survival at 6 months is 81.8% (57/312) for Bio*div*Ysio and 87.9% (37/308) for Duet. By chance, a significantly greater proportion of patients randomized to Bio*div*Ysio had lesions in the LAD (46.1%) compared to Duet (37.7%; $p = 0.02$) as was the proportion of patients receiving more than one stent in the Bio*div*Ysio arm (20% compared with 5.6% for Duet $p = < 0.05$). Subacute stent thrombosis was 0% for the Bio*div*Ysio arm and 0.6% (2/309, $p = $ NS) for the Duet. Multivariate analysis showed that LAD location was a statistically significant factor ($p = 0.03$) for TVF. DISTINCT demonstrates equivalence between a stainless steel stent with a biological coating and a contemporary slotted tube stainless steel stent in patients undergoing percutaneous coronary intervention. These data suggest that the PC Technology coating is safe and benign. The Bio*div*Ysio stent may be valuable when the risk of thrombus is thought to be high.

References

1. Yianni YP. Biocompatibles surfaces based upon biomembrane mimicry. In: Quinn PJ, Cherry RJ (Eds), *Structural and Dynamic Properties of Lipids and Membranes*. Portland Press Research Monograph 1992; 187–216.

2. von Segesser LK, Tonz M, Leskosek B, Turina M. Evaluation of phopholipidic surface coatings ex-vivo. *Int J Artif Organs* 1994;**17**:294–300.

3. Hunter S, Angelini GD. Phosphorylcholine coated chest tubes improve drainage after open heart surgery. *Ann Thoracic Surg* 1993;**56**:1339–42.

4. Chronos NAF, Robinson KA, Kelly AB *et al*. Thromboresistant phosphorylcholine coating for coronary stents. *Eur Heart J* 1997;**18** (suppl 1):52.

5. Malik N, Gunn J, Newman C *et al*. Phosphorylcholine-coated stents: angiographic and morphometric assessment in porcine coronary arteries. *J Am Coll Cardiol* 1998;**31**:411.

6. Van Beusekom HMM, Whelan DM, Krabbendam SC *et al*. Biocompatibility of phosphorylcholine coated stents in a porcine coronary artery model. *Circulation* 1997;**96**(suppl I): 21.

7. Kuiper KK, Robinson KA, Chronos NAF *et al*. Implantation of metal phosphorylcholine coated stents in rabbit iliac and porcine coronary arteries. *Circulation* 1997;**96**(suppl):I–21.

8. Cumberland D, Bonnier H, Colombo A, Fajadet J, Seth A, Cribier A, Wales C. For participants in the divYsio Stent Registry. Phosphorylcholine (PC) coated DivYsio stent-Initial clinical experience from an open registry. *J Am Coll Cardiol* 1998;**31**:407C.

9. Zheng H, Barragan P, Corcos T, Simeoni JB, Favereau X, Roquibert PO, Guerin Y, Sainssous J. Clinical evaluation of a biocompatible phosphorylcholine-coated coronary stent. *J Am Coll Cardiol* 1999;**33**:34A.

10. Armstrong J, Gunn J, Holt CM, Malik N, Rowan L, Stratford P, Cumberland DC. Local drug delivery from coronary stents in the porcine coronary artery. *Heart* 1999;**81**(suppl 1):23A.

11. Boland JL, Corbeij HAM, van der Giessen W *et al* . Multicenter evaluation of the phosphorylcholine-coated stent in BiodivYsio short de novo coronary lesions: The SOPHOS study. *Int J Cardiovasc Intervent* 2000;**3**:215–25.

12. Galli M, Bartonelli A, Bedogni F *et al*. Italian BiodivYsio Open Registry (BiodivYsio PC-Coated Stent): Study of Clinical Outcomes of the Implant of PC-Coated Coronary Stent. *J Invasive Cardiol* 2000;**9**:452–8.

13. Zheng H, Barragan P, Corcos T *et al*. Clinical experience with a new Biocompatible phosphorylcholine-coated coronary stent. *J Invasive Cardiol* 1999;**11**:608–14.

14. Kuiper KKJ, Nordehaug JE. Early mobilisation after protamine reversal of heparin following implantation of phosphorycholine-coated stents in totally occluded coronary arteries. *Am J Cardiol* 2000;**85**:698–702.

15. Feit F, Buller C, Moussa I *et al*. The first prospective randomized comparison of a coronary stent with a synthetic biologic coating compared to a standard stainless steel stent. In preparation.

6. THE Bx VELOCITY™ STENT

Cordis, a Johnson & Johnson Company, Warren, NJ, USA

David R Fischell, Tim A Fischell and Robert E Fischell

Description	
	• Balloon expandable closed cell design
	• BX design permits independent tailoring of radial strength and flexibility elements for optimal stent performance
	• 'N' shaped 'Flex Segment' between stent struts provides optimal flexibility with a completely connected tubular slotted design
	• Full range of sizes in both over-the-wire and rapid exchange configurations
	• Excellent side branch access without strut breakage or loss of vessel scaffolding
	• Wall thickness of 0.0055 inch provides high radial strength and good radiopacity
	• Crimped on low profile matched balloons to create a smooth outer surface for direct stenting
	• 16 atm rated burst pressure, mean burst >20 atm
	• Less than 1.5 mm foreshortening on expansion due to stretch-ability of Flex Segment links.

History	
	• May 1997, first Bx human implants in Milan, Italy
	• 1998–1999, further design improvements resulting in the Bx VELOCITY™ stent
	• January 1999, first human implants of Bx VELOCITY™ stents in Toulouse, France and Milan, Italy
	• May 2000, US launch of OTW Bx VELOCITY™ stent
	• 2000, VENUS study in US demonstrates historically low 6 month TLR (4.6%), 6 month MACE (7.6%) and low SAT (1/304, 0.3%)[1]
	• 2000, coated Bx VELOCITY™ stents: Bx Hepacoat™ is first FDA approved drug-coated stent. Pilot trial of Sirolimus coated Bx VELOCITY™ has zero incidence of restenosis at 1 year

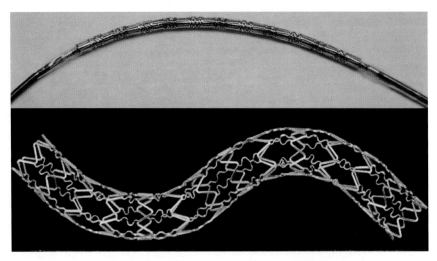

Figure 6.1: *Photographs of the* Bx VELOCITY™ *stent before and after expansion.*

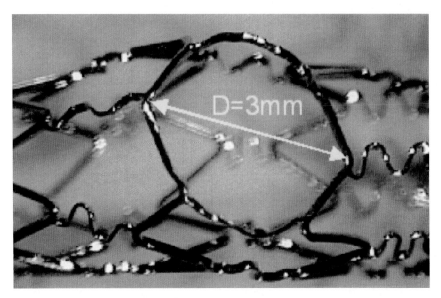

Figure 6.2: *Photograph of the* Bx VELOCITY™ *stent showing the capability for 3 mm side branch access.*

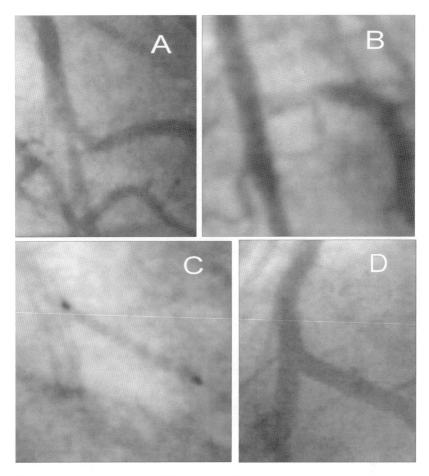

Figure 6.3: Bx VELOCITY™ *treatment of bifurcation, side branch lesion. Pre-intervention angiogram is shown in (a). In (b) main vessel is stented with a* Bx VELOCITY™ *side branch treated with balloon angioplasty with a dissection. In (c), a second* Bx VELOCITY™ *stent is passed through an undilated side cell of main vessel stent without difficulty. T-stenting final result, after deployment of second BX stent, is shown (d).*

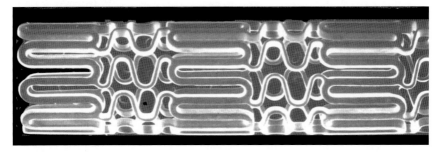

Figure 6.4: *Electron microscope image of the* Bx VELOCITY™ *stent.*

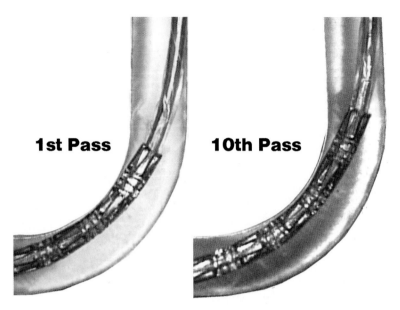

Figure 6.5: *Even after 10 passes through a tight bend, the end of the*
Bx VELOCITY™ *stent remains tightly crimped onto the balloon creating a 'low*
effective profile'.

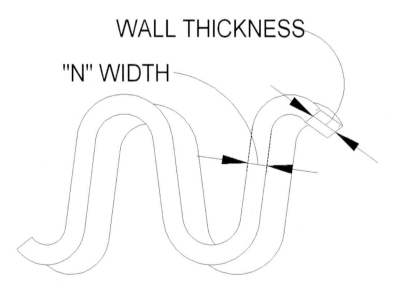

Figure 6.6: *'N' shaped Flex Segment has thin width to allow the stent to flex and*
wall thickness of 0.0055 inch to prevent plaque prolapse.

The Bx VELOCITY™ coronary stent technical specification

Material composition:	316L stainless steel
Degree of radiopacity (grade):	Moderate/high
Ferromagnetism:	Non-ferromagnetic (MRI safe)
Metallic surface area:	<20%
Stent/strut design:	Struts made of curved sections joining negative angle diagonals interconnected with 'N' haped Flex Segments
Strut dimensions:	0.0055 inch wall thickness 0.0052 inch strut width
Profile on delivery system:	<3.2 Fr for 2.25 to 3.0 mm diameter
Longitudinal flexibility:	High
Radial force:	High
Degree of recoil (shape memory):	Minimal
Side branch access:	Excellent (see Figures 6.2 and 6.3)
Total shortening on expansion:	<1.5 mm on all stents up to 4 mm diameter
Currently available diameters:	2.25, 2,5, 2.75, 3.0, 3.5,4.0, 4.5 and 5.0 mm
Currently available lengths:	8, 13, 18, 23, 28 and 33 mm
Recrossability of implanted stents:	Excellent
Drug coatings:	Hepacoat™ covalently bound heparin Sirolimus™ cytostatic antiproliferative
Other non-coronary types available:	Palmaz™ Genesis™ family of peripheral stents

The Bx VELOCITY™ stent delivery system

Mechanism of deployment:	Balloon expandable
Minimal recommended guiding catheter:	6 Fr for 2.25 to 4.5 mm diameter
	7 Fr for 5 mm diameter
Balloon types:	Rapid exchange and over-the-wire
Balloon characteristics:	High pressure semi-compliant
Balloon material:	Duralyn
Offered as a bare stent:	No
Protective sheath	No
Nominal size/quarter size pressures	10 atm/16 atm for most sizes
Rated burst pressure of balloon:	16 atm
Delivery profile:	<3.2 Fr for 2.25 to 3.0 mm
	<4 Fr for 3.5 to 4 mm
	<4 Fr for4.5 to 5 mm
Longitudinal flexibility:	High
Stent retention:	Extremely high
Sizing diameter:	2.25 to 5.0 mm
Recrossability of implanted stents:	Excellent

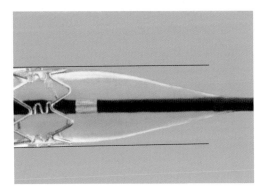

Figure 6.7: Anti-dogboning nature of Bx VELOCITY™ stent delivery system reduces the probability of edge dissections.

Indications for clinical use

- Direct (primary) stenting
- Tortuous anatomy
- Restenotic lesions
- Ostial lesions
- Lesions on a bend
- Placement into a side branch
- Acute closure and bailout situations*
- Total occlusions
- De novo lesions*
- Acute MI (Hepacoat™)
- Sub-optimal PTCA
- Patients with allergies or contraindications for clopidigrel and ticlopidine (Hepacoat™)*

* FDA approved indications

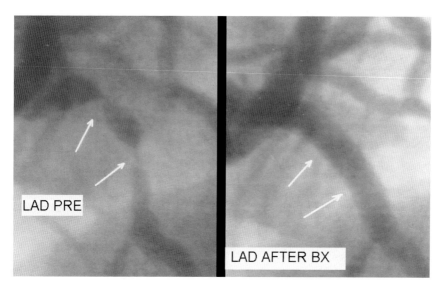

Figure 6.8: *Acute result with* Bx VELOCITY™ *Stent. Left: tandem high-grade lesions of proximal LAD. Right: acute results following direct stenting with a 3.5 mm* Bx VELOCITY™ *stent — note smooth edges, minimal residual stenosis and to vessel contour.*

Why I like my stent

The Bx VELOCITY™ stent with its fully connected design and low profile delivery system provides clinicians with the most desired attributes in a stent.

1. Flexibility, low profile, smooth outer surface and superb stent retention to enable direct stenting of most lesions.
2. Radial strength to provide a large post-procedural lumen with minimal recoil and vessel wall injury[3] – the best predictor of the patient's late vessel patency. (Final average MLD in VENUS Study[1] of 1.8%.)
3. 6, 7 or 9 cells around optimizes stent performance at all diameters and provides good vessel wall coverage.
4. 16 atm rated burst pressure stent delivery system.
5. While most stents oversize 10% between the nominal and rated burst balloon pressures, the Bx VELOCITY™ oversizes exactly 0.25 mm for most sizes.
6. 6 French guide compatibility up to 4.5 mm diameter devices.
7. 5.5 mm wall thickness for radial strength and good radiopacity.
8. A full range of diameters and lengths in both over-the-wire and rapid exchange designs.
9. 'N' shaped flex segments provide excellent vessel conformability and kids-branch access with excellent scaffolding.

The Bx VELOCITY™ stent has also been designed to provide an excellent platform for drug coatings including Hepacoat™ and Sirolimus.

The Cordis Bx VELOCITY™ stent is an example of the application of clinical input, science and engineering to create a nearly optimal stent design.

Drug coatings on the Bx VELOCITY™ stent

The Bx VELOCITY™ stent is now available with the Hepacoat™ (see Figure 6.8) covalently bonded heparin coating to reduce the probability of subacute or late thrombosis. In the Benestent II and TOSCA studies the Hepacoat™ coating on Palmaz-Schatz stents had only one incidence of sub-acute thrombosis in 817 elective stent implants (0.012%).[4,5]

The Bx VELOCITY™ is now in randomized clinical trials with a Sirolimus antiproliferative coating. In the pilot study of 30 cases reported by Sousa and Serruys there were no restenoses, no TLRs and a late loss at 1 year of ~0.1 mm diameter.[6] Figure 6.9 shows the pre-immediate post- and 1-year angiograms of one of these cases.

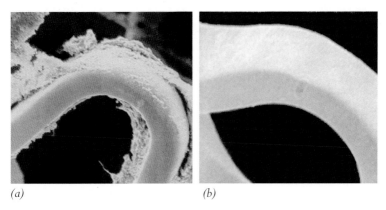

(a)   (b)

Figure 6.9: *Scanning electron micrographs of uncoated (a) and Hepacoat™ coated (b) Bx VELOCITY™ stents 2 hours after implant. Note the platelet deposition on the uncoated stent and pristine appearance of the Hepacoat™ stent.*

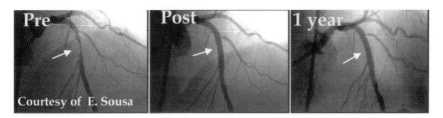

Figure 6.10: *Pre-procedure, post-procedure and 1 year follow up of Sirolimus-coated Bx VELOCITY™ stent implanted in a human coronary artery.*

References

1. Zidar JP, Fry E, Lambert C, Rubinstein R, Raizner AE, Fischell TA, Janzer S, Popma JI, Kuntz RE. The VENUS trial: a multicenter registry of the Cordis BX *VELOCITY*™ stent. [abstract] *Am J Cardiol* 2000; TCT Supplement **86**(Suppl 8A): 171.

2. Carter AJ, Scott D, Rahdert D, Bailey L, De Vries J, Ayerdi K, Turnland T, Jones R, Vinnani R, Fischell TA. Computer assisted stent design favorably influences the arterial response in normal porcine coronary arteries. *J Invasive Cardiol* 1999; **11**:127–34.

3. Carter AJ, Scott D, Bailey L, Devries J, Ayerdi K, Fischell DR, Fischell RE, Turnland T, Jones R, Virmani R. Fischell TA. Stent design: in the 'ends' it matter [abstract]. *Circulation* 1997; **96**:1–8.

4. Serruys PW, van Hout B, Bonnier H, Legrand V, Garcia E, Macaya C, Sousa E, van der Giessen W, Colombo A. Seabra-Gomes R, Kiemeneij F, Ruygrok P, Ormiston J, Emanuelsson H, Fajadet J, Haude M, Klugmann S, Morel MA. Randomised comparison of implantation of heparin-coated stents with balloon angioplasty in selected patients with coronary artery disease (Benestent ll). *Lancet* 1998; **352**:673–81.

5. Buller CE, Dzavik V, Carere RG, Mancini GB, Barbeau G, Lazzam C, Anderson TJ, Kundtson ML, Marquis JF, Suzuki T, Cohen EA, Fox RS, Teo KK. Primary stenting versus balloon angioplasty in occluded coronary arteries: the total occlusion study of Canada (TOSCA). *Circulation* 1999; **100**:236–42.

6. Sousa JE, Costa MA, Abizaid A, Abizaid AS, Feres F, Pinto I, Seixas AC, Staico R, Mattos LA, Sousa A, Falotico, R, Jaeger J, Popma JJ, Serruys PW. Lack of Neointimal proliferation after implantation of sirolimus-coated stents in human coronary arteries. A quantitative coronary angiography and three-dimensional intravascular ultrasound study. *Circulation* 2001; **103**:192–5.

7. THE CARBOSTENT SIRIUS STENT

Sorin Biomedica S.p.A., Saluggia (VC), Italy

Antonio Colombo and Takuro Takagi

Description	• Balloon expandable laser cut 316 LVM high grade pure stainless steel stent (VM: vacuum melted) • Tubular stent with homogenous multicellular architecture • Integral and permanent coating of pure turbostratic carbon (Carbofilm™). Turbostratic refers to the specific crystal structure of the carbon atoms

Brief history of the stent	• 1960, development of pyrolytic carbon for applications in the nuclear energy field. Since the late 1960s it has been used for components of cardiac valve prostheses because of its superior bio- and hemocompatibility and thromboresistance. Pyrolysis is the process used to obtain turbostratic carbon by lysis of hydrocarbons at very high temperatures. • 1982, development at Sorin Biomedica of a low temperature process for the deposition of thin films of turbostratic carbon (Carbofilm™) on metals and polymers used for implantable prostheses. • 1998, first clinical experience and approval for marketing of Carbostent (Dr Antonio Bartorelli and Dr David Antoniucci). • 2000, first clinical experience published by Dr Antoniucci et al.[1]

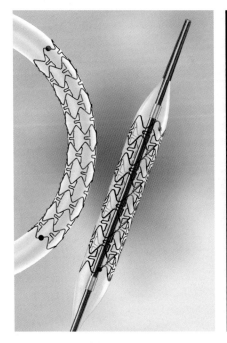

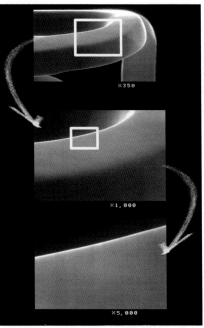

Figure 7.1: *The Sorin Carbostent on the balloon after expansion and in a curved condition. Notice the absence of a 'fish scale effect' and the stent radiopaque markers at the ends.*

Figure 7.2: *Magnification of the mirror-like surface of the Carbostent.*

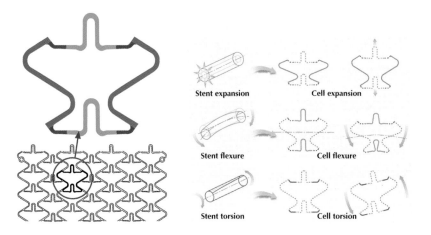

Figure 7.3: *The Carbostent cell consists of different curved segments, each one designed with a variable cross-section to optimize the individual mechanical response to stent expansion, flexure and torsion.*

50

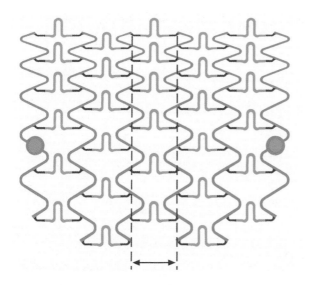

Figure 7.4: *Flat layout of the Carbostent during expansion. The ends of the omega elements remain aligned, preserving the original stent length.*

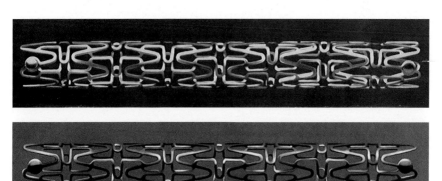

Figure 7.5: *The Carbostent before (top panel) and after (bottom panel) Carbofilm™ coating.*

Carbostent SIRIUS technical specifications

Material composition:	316 LVM stainless steel
Degree of radiopacity (grade):	Low; there are platinum markers at stent ends
Ferromagnetism:	Non-ferromagnetic
MRI:	MRI-safe
Metallic surface area (metal: artery, expanded):	12–17%
Stent design:	Laser micromachined tube, multicellular architecture with curved segment of variable cross-section
Coatings:	Permanent and integral film (0.3–0.5 µm) of turbostratic carbon (Carbofirm™)
Radiopaque markers:	Two terminal platinum markers (350 µm)
Strut dimensions:	0.003 inch (0.075 mm)
Strut width:	0.003–0.005 inch (0.075–0.125 mm)
Longitudinal flexibility:	High
Percentage shortening on expansion:	0%
Degree of recoil (shape memory):	3–6%
Currently available diameters (only mounted):	2.5 mm (4 cells) 3.0–3.5 mm (5 cells) 4.0 mm (6 cells)
Currently available lengths	9, 12, 15, 19, 25 mm
Recrossability of implanted stent	Good
Other non-coronary types available:	None

Carbostent SIRIUS delivery system

Mechanism of deployment:	Balloon expandable
Protective sheath:	No
Design:	Rapid exchange
Balloon characteristics:	Semi-compliant, 0.5 mm distal and proximal hangover
Position of radio-opaque markers:	Two on the balloon, denoting proximal and distal stent ends
Rated burst pressure of balloon:	16 atm
Average burst pressure of balloon:	22 atm
Guidewire compatibility:	0.014 inch (0.36 mm)
Minimum internal diameter of guide catheter:	5Fr
Offered as a bare stent:	No

Tips and tricks for delivery

This stent is quite flexible, smooth, and well secured on the balloon, complex anatomy is not usually a problem. When the lesion characteristics do not suggest the need for predilatation, direct stenting is feasible. The balloon is semi-compliant (3.5 mm balloon will grow to 3.88 mm when inflated at 16 atm) and has limited hangover. Normally 12 atm is sufficient to expand the stent, but this is quite dependent on the characteristics of the lesion. In case of a hard or calcified lesion, consider using a short, non-compliant balloon to expand the stent fully in order to avoid distal or proximal trauma or dissections.

Indications for use

Elective treatment for occlusive lesions of native coronaries and venous or arterial bypass grafts. Bailout use for unfavorable results of PTCA.

Why I like my stent

- The stent is flexible due to the design and to the thin metal, and has a good coverage of the lesion site
- The stent has good side branch access and with an additional balloon the cell can be enlarged to 11.0 mm^2 in surface area
- The presence of two visible platinum end markers makes positioning and post-dilatation safe and reliable
- There are multiple lengths and sizes. The number of stent cells changes according to the stent size: 2.5 mm (four cells), 3.0–3.5 mm (five cells), 4.0 mm (six cells). This means that for small vessels the amount of metal is someway proportionally reduced
- The animal data[2] and some preliminary human registry data[1,3,4] show a reduced thrombogenicity. This feature is currently being tested in a randomized trial (SAFE trial: SORIN and Aspirin Following Elective stenting).

Design characteristics

The Sorin Carbostent has an original cellular geometry designed to match the ideal functional features of an implantable stent to the different lesion characteristics present in coronary artery disease. Each cell of the Carbostent is an elemental structure that realizes a full, self-contained mechanical functionality. The cell consists of different curved segments, each one designed with variable cross-section to optimize the individual mechanical response to stent expansion, flexure and torsion (Figure 7.3). The aim is to avoid stress concentration and elastic distortion that may stimulate abnormal cell proliferation, and to create a good elastic matching between the stent structure and the vascular coronary tissue. The stent cells are connected at the mid-point of the expanding segments (Figure 7.4): the advantage deriving from this cell interconnection scheme is to realize minimal longitudinal shortening of the stent upon expansion. The stent has a versatile range of sizes. The lengths are 9, 12, 15, 19 and 25 mm, available in the 2.5 mm nominal diameter (four cells configuration), 3.0–3.5 mm (five cells), and 4.0 mm (six cells). Two radiopaque terminal platinum markers, positioned at the stent ends, ensure excellent fluoroscopic visibility without interfering with the angiographic appearance and QCA analysis of the contrast-filled coronary lumen. The entire surface of the Carbostent undergoes electrochemical treatment and mirror-like polishing derived from Sorin's heart valve technologies, that provide round edges and a smooth strut surface (Figure 7.2). These features enhance stent trackability (friction-less surface) and minimize the risk of injury to the vessel wall (round edges).

Carbofilm™ coating

The Carbostent is integrally coated with a permanent thin film (0.3–0.5 μm) of turbostratic carbon (Carbofilm™), which, when applied to cardiac valves renders the surface thromboresistant and enhances biocompatibility (Figure 7.5). Carbofilm™ consists of pure carbon characterized by a polycrystalline structure substantially identical to that of pyrolytic carbon. The bulk pyrolytic carbon manufacturing process, developed by Sorin Biomedica in the early 1960s when the company was a nuclear research center, has been used worldwide for more than 30 years in the production of the most critical cardiovascular prostheses, the mechanical heart valves. Pyrolytic carbon is an ideal material for prostheses in contact with blood because of its unique physical and chemical characteristics, such as chemical inertness, isotropy, low weight, compactness, elasticity and high strength.[6–8] These properties are accompanied by great hardness and wear resistance.[9] The hemocompatibilty of a pyrolytic carbon-covered prosthesis is largely dependent on atraumatic interaction with the proteins that form a layer adhering to the pyrolytic carbon surface, without altering their structure.[10–13] The pyrolytic carbon process involves a high temperature, which precludes the possibility of coating most materials, including stainless steel. In 1982, Sorin Biomedica's laboratories developed an original room temperature process for the deposition of thin films of turbostratic carbon (Carbofilm™) on a variety of substrates (metals, polymers). This is done in a high vacuum to prevent chemical reactions, preserve the purity of the deposited material, and retain all chemical, physical and biological properties of pyrolytic carbon.[1] This technique obtains intrinsically stable bonds, resulting in permanent adhesion of the coating to the substrate – even after very long exposure to blood – and provides an extremely thin film (0.3–0.5 μm), which does not alter the morphologic and physical characteristics of the coated substrate. Extensive laboratory and in vivo studies conducted on Carbofilm™ coated vascular prostheses have shown reduced thrombus formation, platelet adhesion and activation.[14–17] Moreover, a tissue reaction characterized by a well-organized neointima, devoid of foreign body giant cells and significantly thinner than controls, has consistently been observed.[18] The flexibility of Sorin's coating technique allowed the CarbofilmTM to be applied to a variety of materials currently used for implantable devices: titanium alloy for valve housings, polyester fabric for vascular grafts, silicone rubber for pacemaker leads, and, more recently, stainless steel for the Carbostent.

55

Examples illustrating pre- and post-Carbostent implantation (Figures 7.6–7.8)

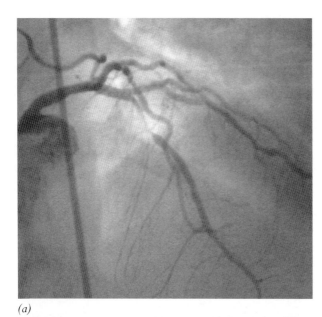

(a)

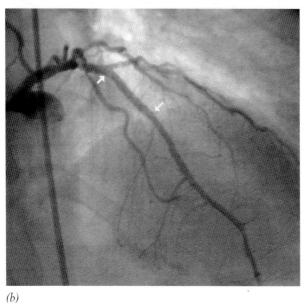

(b)

Figure 7.6:
Example of precise stent placement very close to bifurcation site without plaque shift to the bifurcation. (a) A critical de novo stenosis of mid-anterior descending artery in a 53-year-old female with stable angina. Notice the lesion extends to bifurcation of diagonal branch. (b) After stent implantation. Marker at stent edge enabled to adequate positioning. Arrows indicate markers.

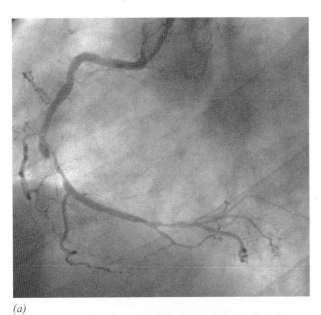

(a)

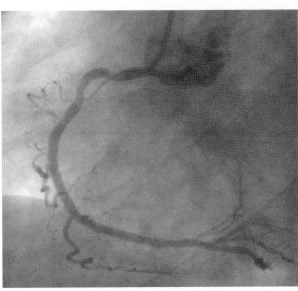

(b)

Figure 7.7:
Example of stenting
an unstable plaque.
(a) An eccentric
stenosis with
ulceration is seen in
the mid-right
coronary artery in a
57-year-old male
with new onset
unstable angina. (b)
Angiographic result
after treatment with
25 mm long
Carbostent SIRIUS
demonstrating smooth
in-stent lumen.

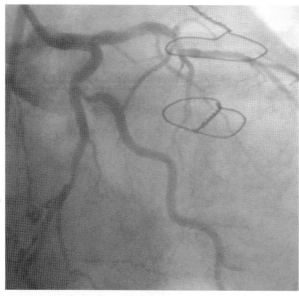

(a)

Figure 7.8:
Example of stent placement in a tortuous vessel. (a) An ostial stenosis in obtuse marginal branch in a 70-year-old male with stable angina. Notice severe tortuosity of the circumflex artery. (b) Result after successful deployment of 12 mm length Carbostent SIRIUS.

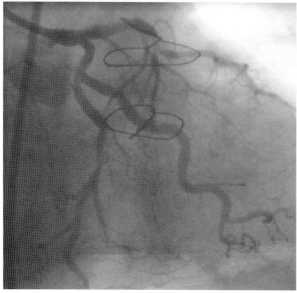

(b)

Intravascular ultrasound: 2-D and 3–D (Figures 7.9 and 7.10)

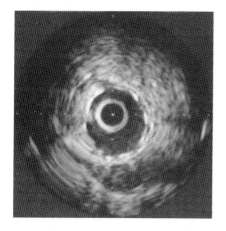

Figure 7.9: 2–D image after implantation of Carbostent SIRIUS. Good apposition and circular expansion of the stent can be seen.

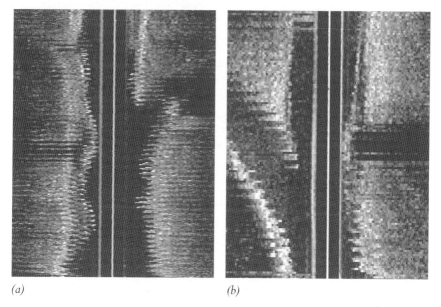

(a)   *(b)*

Figure 7.10: Free access to a side branch. (a) 3–D intravascular ultrasound image after deployment of 15 mm long stent to anterior descending artery (LAD). This image was reconstructed with pullback through LAD. Diagonal branch can be seen inside the stent. (b) Pullback through diagonal branch to LAD, no protrusion of stent strut can be seen.

On-going or planned trials

Name	Purpose	Patients	Type of trial	Number of sites	Status follow up	Results
ANTARES	Preliminary evaluation of Carbostent thromboresistance ASA only	110	Registry	1 in Italy	Complete 30 days clinical data available; paper in press	Thrombosis rate: 0%
HURRICANE	Patient at high risk of restenosis	112	Registry	1 in Italy	Complete 6 months angiographic data available; paper in press	Restenosis rate: 26% and loss index 0.35
ACE	1 and 6 months MACE of Carbostent with or without abciximab in ACS	200	Randomized	2 in Italy 1 in Germany 1 in Argentina	In progress	
SAFE	Thromboresistant properties of Carbostent at low antiplatelet regimen ASA only vs ASA + thienopyridine	1400	Randomized	15–18 in Italy	In progress	
CARBOSTENT	6 months stent restenosis of Carbostent vs. Medtronic AVE S670 and S7	410	Randomized	20 in Europe	In progress	
SIROCCO	6 months stent restenosis by IVUS of Carbostent and Multilink Tetra	70	Randomized	2 in France	Awaiting to start	
SESAME	6 months stent restenosis of Carbostent vs. POBA in small vessels	610	Randomized	16 in Europe	Awaiting start	

Review of the current published literature

Antoniucci et al.[1] reported initial experience with Sorin Carbostent in a prospective registry of 112 patients who underwent stent implantation for treatment of 132 lesions from April 1998 through January 1999. The purpose of this study was to evaluate the immediate and long-term clinical and angiographic outcome after Carbostent implantation in patients with coronary artery disease in native vessels. Patients with stable and unstable angina were included for elective and bailout stenting indications. The following lesions were excluded from the study: previously stented lesions, acute myocardial infarction, and lesions with a reference diameter <2.5 mm The mean age of the patients was 61 years; 82% were male, 16% were diabetics, 55% had prior MI, and 38% had multivessel disease. Forty-seven per cent of the lesions were in the left anterior descending location, 39% in the right coronary artery and 13% in the circumflex artery. According to the ACC/AHA lesion classification, 38% of lesions were type B2 and C, lesion length was >15 mm in 29%, and a chronic total occlusion was present in 8%.

All patients were treated with aspirin (300 mg) and ticlopidine (500 mg per day) for 1 month, no patient received GPIIb/IIIa antagonists. Procedural data revealed a balloon-to-artery ratio for final stent dilatation of 1.0, and an average final dilatation pressure of 15 atm. Delivery success was achieved in all attempted cases.

Angiographic follow-up was available in 96% of the patients at 6 months. The early and late outcomes are shown in the tables. The event-free survival rate was 84%. The angiographic and clinical results with the Carbostent were promising, despite the unfavorable clinical and angiographic characteristics of patients enrolled. The relatively low late loss that was found on follow-up could be a reflection of the high biocompatibility of this stent, although the large mean reference diameter could also explain the low restenosis rate.

Combined antiplatelet therapy, advances in stent technology and the procedure (optimal stent implantation) reduced the frequency of thrombotic complications. However, the introduction of new technologies such as brachytherapy and some drug eluting stents seems to have introduced the problem of stent thrombosis. Delayed endothelialization caused by these antiproliferative approaches is a possible mechanism for this event. The availability of a true non-thrombogenic stent therefore becomes a real issue. Theoretical reasons, laboratory data and preliminary clinical results all support a lower thrombogenicity for this carbon-coated stent. The need for hard clinical data to confirm these expectations will be addressed by ongoing clinical trials.

The Carbostent thromboresistance was first assessed by Bartorelli, who obtained a 0% thrombosis (at 30 days and 6 months) with the ANTARES pilot study (*Cathet Cardiovasc Interven*; in press) where 110 patients, implanted with Carbostent, were treated only with aspirin as the sole antiplatelet regimen. Clinical information of these encouraging results is being sought in the SAFE trial, that has been designed as a two arm randomized, prospective evaluation in 1400 patients submitted to the conventional aspirin plus ticlopidine or aspirin alone antiplatelet treatments. The aim of the SAFE study is to confirm that the acute and subacute thrombosis rate of the two patient subsets is the same, confirming the ANTARES results and supporting the safety of Carbostent implantation even with a low dosage antiplatelet regimen.

Possible advantages of carbon coating may also apply to patients who show allergy to nickel or other metals usually present in small amounts in stainless steel.[19]

Clinical outcomes

	0–30 days (n = 112)	31–180 days (n = 112)
Any adverse event*	1 (1%)	12 (11%)
Death	0	1 (1%)
Q wave MI	0	0
Non-Q wave MI	1 (1%)	0
TVR	0	11 (10%)
Thrombosis	0	0

*Death, MI or TVR (MI, myocardial infarction; TVR, target vessel revascularization).

Angiographic outcomes

Preprocedural QCA (n = 132)	
Reference diameter, mm	3.33 ± 0.49
MLD, mm	0.70 ± 0.42
Percent stenosis	79 ± 12 %
Lesion length, mm	12.5 ± 7.0
Postprocedural QCA (n = 132)	
Reference diameter, mm	3.39 ± 0.46
MLD, mm	3.26 ± 0.45
Percent stenosis	4 ± 7%
Acute gain, mm	2.56 ± 0.58
Six-month follow-up QCA (n = 127)	
Reference diameter, mm	3.27 ± 0.46
MLD, mm	2.53 ± 0.82
Per cent stenosis	22 ± 23 %
Late loss, mm	0.75 ± 0.73
Net gain, mm	1.82 ± 0.83
Loss index	0.29 ± 0.28
Six-month follow-up angiographic outcomes (n = 127)	
Binary (>50%) restenosis	14 (11%)

QCA: quantitative coronary angiography; MLD: minimal lumen diameter.

References

1. Antoniucci D, Bartorelli A, Valenti R, Montorsi P, Santoro GM, Fabbiocchi F, Bolognese L, Loaldi A, Trapani M, Trabattoni D, Moschi G, Galli S. Clinical and angiographic outcome after coronary arterial stenting with the carbostent. *Am J Cardiol* 2000; **85**:821–5.

2. Virmani R, Santarelli A, Galloni M *et al*. Tissue response and biocompatibility of the Sorin Carbostent: experimental results in porcine coronary arteries. *Am J Cardiol* 1998; **82**(Suppl 7A):65.

3. Antoniucci D, Valenti R, Moschi G *et al*. Clinical and angiographic outcome after coronary arterial stenting with the Carbostent in patients at high risk for restenosis (the Second Carbostent Registry). *Am J Cardiol* 2000; **86**(Suppl 8A):17i.

4. Bartorelli AL, Fabbiocchi F, Montorsi P *et al*. Aspirin-alone treatment after Carbostent stenting: the ANTARES study. *Am J Cardiol* 2000; **86**(Suppl 8A):18i.

5. Kaae JL, Gulden TD. Structure and mechanical properties of co-deposited pyrolytic C-SiC alloys. *J Am Ceram Soc*1971; **54**:605–9.

6. Bokros JC. Variation in the crystallinity of carbon deposited in fluidized beds. *Biomat Med Dev Art Org* 1965; **3**:201–11.

7. Shim HS. The behavior of isotropic pyrolytic carbon under cyclic loading. *Biomat Med Dev Art Org* 1974; **2**:55–65.

8. Shim HS. The wear of titanium alloy, and UHMW polyethylene caused by LTI carbon stellite 21. *J Bioeng* 1977; **1**:223–9.

9. Bokros JC. Carbon biomedical devices. *Carbon* 1977; **15**:355–71.

10. Haubold AD. Blood/carbon interaction. *ASAIO J* 1983; **6**:88–92.

11. Benson J. Elemental carbon as a biomaterial. *J Biomed Master Res Symp* 1971; **2**:41–7.

12. Haubold AD, Shim HS, Bokros JC. Biocompatibility of clinical implant materials. In: *Carbon in Medical Devices*, 1981. Williams DF, ed., Boca Raton, USA.

13. Paccagnella A, Majni G, Ottaviani G *et al*. Properties of a new carbon film for biomedical applications. *J Art Org* 1986; **9**:127–33.

14. Sbarbati R, Giannessi D, Cenni MC *et al*. Pyrolytic carbon coating enhances teflon and dacron fabric compatibility with endothelial cell growth. *Int J Art Organs* 1991; **14**:491–8.

15. Cenni E, Granchi D, Arciola CR *et al*. Platelet and coagulation factor variations induced in vitro by polyethylene terephtalate (Dacron) coated with pyrolytic carbon. *Biomaterials* 1995; **16**:973–6.

16. Cenni E, Granchi D, Arciola CR *et al*. Adhesive protein expression on endothelial cells after contact in vitro with polyethylene terephtalate coated with pyrolytic carbon. *Biomaterials* 1995; **16**:1223–7.

17. Cenni E, Granchi D, Ciapetti G *et al*. In vitro complement activation after contact with pyrolytic carbon-coated and uncoated polyethylene terephthalate. *J Mat Sci: Materials in Medicine* 1997; **8**:771–4.

18. Aebischer P, Goodard M, Hunter TJ *et al*. Tissue reaction to fabrics coated with turbostratic carbon: subcutaneous versus vascular implants. *Biomaterials* 1998; **9**:80–85.

19. Koster R, Vieluf D, Kiehn M *et al*. Nickel and molybdenum contact allergies in patients with coronary in-stent restenosis. *Lancet* 2000; **356**:1895–7.

8. THE CORDYNAMIC APOLO STENT

Iberhospitex SA, Barcelona, Spain

Amadeu Betriu, Isabel Pérez, Aniceto López and
Lluis Duocastella

Description	• Segmented multicellular slotted tube with alternating bridge connections
	• Balloon expandable stent
	• Slotted tube type, tubular stent

History	• 1999, CE marked for clinical use
	• 1999–2000, clinical trial in humans
	• 2000–2001, ongoing multicenter registry study of restenosis

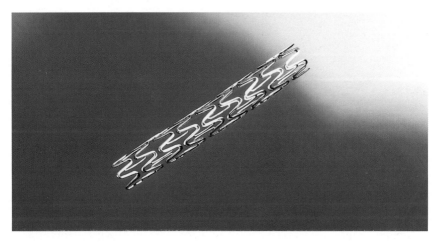

Figure 8.1: *Picture of a loose stent.*

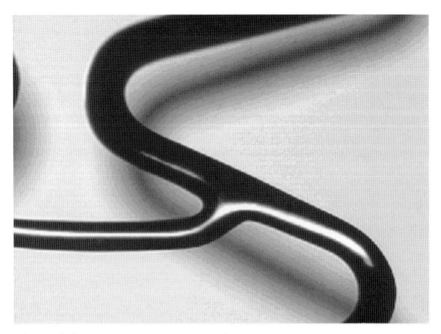

Figure 8.2: *Picture showing the quality of electropolishing..*

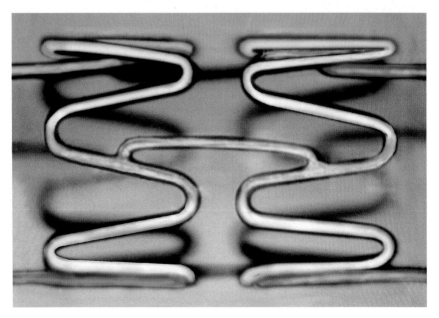

Figure 8.3: *Expanded stent, showing the main structure and the bridge connection.*

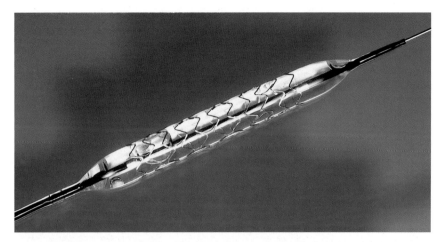

Figure 8.4: Expanded Cordynamic Apolo stent on balloon.

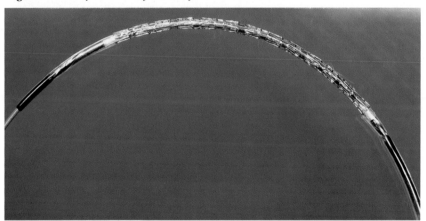

Figure 8.5: Crimped Cordynamic Apolo stent on delivery device.

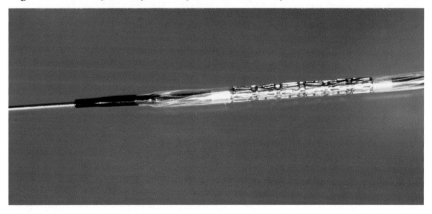

Figure 8.6: Cordynamic stent on delivery device, showing crimped profile and method of securement.

Cordynamic Apolo stent technical specifications

Material composition:	316 LVM stainless steel
Degree of radiopacity:	Moderate
Ferromagnetism:	Non-ferromagnetic
MRI:	Safe
Metallic surface area	
Expanded (18 mm stent):	Diameter 2.5 mm; 20%
	Diameter 3.0 mm; 16.6%
	Diameter 3.5 mm; 14.3%
	Diameter 4.0 mm; 12.5%
	Diameter 4.5 mm; 11.1%
Unexpanded (18 mm stent):	Diameter 1.8 mm; 36.3%
Metallic cross-sectional area:	0.1152 mm^2
Stent design:	Slotted tube stent
Strut design:	Sinus curve, rounded edges
Strut dimensions:	0.0096 mm^2
Strut thickness:	0.115 mm at main area; 0.1 mm at bridge connection
Profile: non-expanded (non-crimped):	1.8 mm
On the balloons:	<1 mm till 3.0 mm balloon about 1 mm from 3.5 to 4.5 mm
Longitudinal flexibility:	High
Percentage shortening on expansion:	<1%
Expansion range:	2 to 5
Currently available diameters:	2.5, 3.0, 3.5, 4.0, 4.5 mm
Currently available lengths:	9, 14, 18, 23, 28, 36 mm
Recrossability of implanted stent:	Excellent

Cordynamic Apolo stent delivery system

Mechanism of deployment:	Balloon expandable
Protective sheath:	No
Monorail system:	Yes
Minimal internal diameter of guiding catheter:	0.056 inch, 5 Fr
Balloon characteristics:	Semicompliant balloon, Hypotube design Balloon folded in four wings to ensure uniform stent deployment
Balloon material:	Nylon
Balloon compliance:	Nominal at 10 atm +0.25 mm at 14 atm Rated burst pressure; 16 atm
Further dilatation recommended:	At physician's discretion
Recommended deployment pressure:	Between 10 and 16 atm
Longitudinal flexibility:	High
Position of radiopaque markers:	At both ends of the stent
Stent security:	The special crimping process ensures the stent retention
Delivery profile:	Less than 1 mm
Offered as bare stent:	Yes

Tips and tricks for delivery

No special tips for delivery. For obtaining the best final result, utilize the two radiopaque markers on the delivery system. The nominal pressure is 10 atmospheres; at 14 atmospheres the stent expands 0.25 mm more than at nominal pressure. The stent is suitable for direct stenting due to its low profile.

71

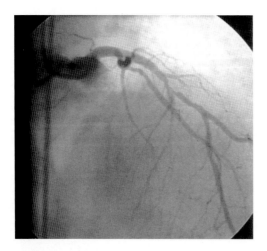

Figure 8.7: *LAD lesion before stent implantation.*

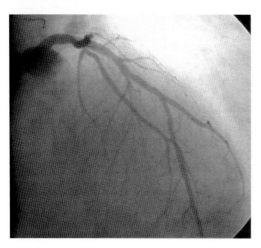

Figure 8.8: *Angiographic result after Cordynamic Apolo stent implantation in LAD.*

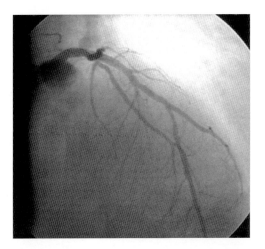

Figure 8.9: *RCA lesion before stent implantation, showing lesion in bifurcation.*

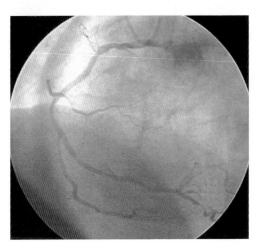

Figure 8.10: *Angiographic result after Cordynamic Apolo stent implantation in RCA.*

Indications for use

- Native coronary lesions
- Restenotic lesions after PTCA
- High risk of restenosis after PTCA
- Acute myocardial infarction
- Dissection after PTCA
- Lesions in tortuous vessels

Why I like my stent

- Due to its design characteristics the stent combines flexibility during delivery with high radial strength after implantation
- Very low crossing profile
- Low deployment pressure, high implantation pressure if required
- Balloon crimping system which ensures retention of the stent

9. The Coroflex and Coroflex Delta Coronary Stent Systems

B Braun Melsungen AG, Berlin, Germany

Nigel M Wheeldon

Description	• The Coroflex Coronary Stent is a laser-cut, 316L stainless steel, balloon-expandable slotted-tube, which has rounded edges and is electropolished.
	• The stent comprises multiple sinusoidal ring elements connected by bridges from their mid-points, an arrangement which allows exceptional flexibility.
	• The Coroflex stent is premounted on the Larus high-pressure, rapid-exchange balloon catheter, which has a very low profile, a scratch-resistant surface and two radiopaque stent position markers.
	• The resulting delivery system combines excellent flexibility with a very low crossing profile and is particularly suited for negotiating tortuous anatomy, or in situations where direct stenting is indicated.

History	• 1998: European safety study
	• 1998–99: International registry
	• 1999: Launch of Coroflex stent delivery system
	• 1999: Completion of prospective, multicentre follow-up study

Coroflex technical specifications

Material composition:	316L stainless steel
Degree of radiopacity:	Low
Ferromagnetism:	Low (MRI safe)
Metallic surface area (metal:artery expanded):	12% (expanded)
Stent design:	Laser-cut, slotted-tube with sinusoidal ring elements joined at their mid-points by flexible bridges
Strut design:	Electropolished, ellipto-rectangular, rounded-edges
Strut thickness:	0.0036 inch (0.09 mm)
Delivery profile (crossing profile):	0.04 inch (0.97 mm)
Longitudinal flexibility:	High
Percentage shortening on expansion:	1–3%
Expansion range:	2.5–4.5 mm
Degree of recoil (shape memory):	4–5%
Radial force:	0.6 atm
Available diameters:	2.5, 3.0, 3.5 and 4.0 mm
Available lengths:	8, 13, 16 and 25 mm (premounted)
Recrossability:	Excellent
Side branch access:	Excellent

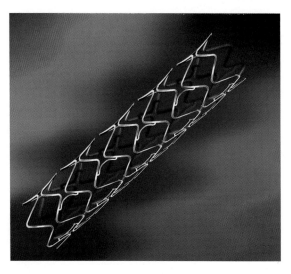

Figure 9.1: The expanded Coroflex stent.

Coroflex Delta technical specifications

Material composition:	316L stainless steel
Degree of radiopacity:	Medium
Ferromagnetism:	Low
Metallic surface area:	14%
Stent design:	Laser cut, slotted-tube with sinusoidal ring elements joined at their mid-points by flexible bridges
Strut design:	Electropolished, ellipto-rectangular, rounded-edges
Strut thickness:	0.0047 inch (0.12 mm)
Delivery profile:	0.042 inch (1.05 mm)
Longitudinal flexibility:	High
Shortening:	1–3%
Expansion range:	2.5–4.5 mm
Recoil:	3–5%
Radial force:	1.5 atm
Diameters:	2.5, 3.0, 3.5, 4.0 mm
Lengths:	8, 13, 16, 25 mm
Recrossability:	Excellent
Side branch access:	Excellent

Coroflex stent delivery system

Mechanism of deployment:	Balloon expandable
Minimal internal diameter of guiding catheter:	Pre-mounted stent 6Fr compatible Larus balloon 5Fr compatible
Premounted on delivery catheter:	Yes
Premounted on high-pressure balloon:	Yes. Larus balloon catheter
Balloon material:	Pamax
Guidewire lumen:	0.014 inch (0.36 mm)
Minimum recommended guide:	6Fr
Protective sheath:	No
Position of radiopaque markers:	Proximal and distal to the stent.
Rated burst pressure of balloon:	15 atm (2.5–3.5 mm) 12 atm (4.0 mm)
Delivery profile:	Very low. Mounted stent profile 0.97 mm
Longitudinal flexibility:	Excellent
Balloon compliance:	Nominal at 6 atm
Recommended deployment pressure:	8–12 atm

Tips and tricks for delivery

- The Coroflex stent delivery system behaves very well such that no specific additional techniques are required for stent deployment. In many instances handling of the stent is similar to that of the balloon alone
- Preparation of the stent balloon is not required. Should balloon preparation be preferred, this can be performed with the stent across the lesion prior to inflation
- The low crossing profile of the system lends itself to lesions suitable for direct stenting and the delivery balloon has the capacity for high-pressure inflation should this be required
- Stent deployment occurs at low pressures (4 bar) and the stent is often optimally deployed at 8 bar, although higher pressures may be required depending on vessel size
- Shortening is minimal and side branch access is good

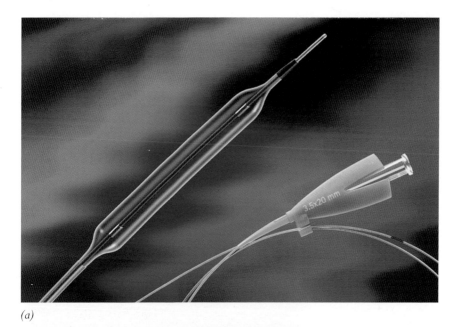

(a)

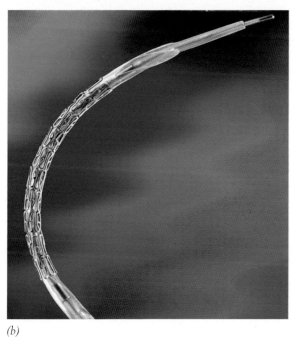

(b)

Figure 9.2: (a) The Larus balloon catheter; (b) The Coroflex stent delivery system.

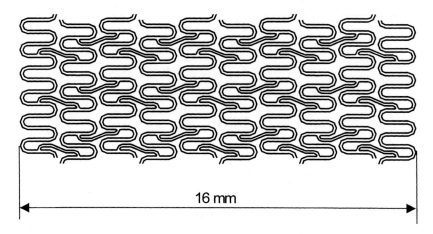

16 mm

Figure 9.3: *Technical drawing of Coroflex stent design.*

Indications for use

- De novo and restenotic lesions in native coronary arteries or where suboptimal results due to dissection or recoil occur
- Particularly useful in tortuous anatomy where flexibility is important
- Likely to have a role in direct stenting in view of very low crossing profile

Why I like the Coroflex stent

- Excellent flexibility, trackability and low crossing profile
- Balloon-like handling characteristics
- Compatibility with 6Fr guiding catheters
- Low-profile, pre-mounted, rapid-exchange delivery system
- Two balloon markers for accurate stent positioning
- Low deployment pressure although high-pressure balloon capability if required
- Low radiopacity resulting in good vessel visualization after deployment
- Suitable for direct stenting of appropriate lesions

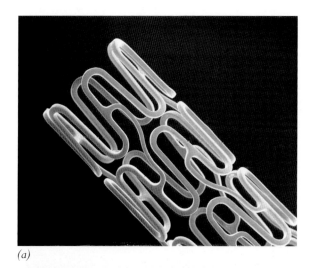

Figure 9.4(a–c):
Scanning electron
micrographs of Coroflex
coronary stent design

(a)

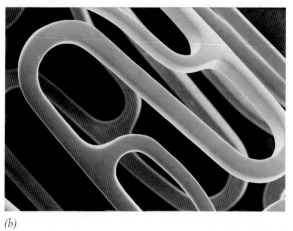

(b)

(c)

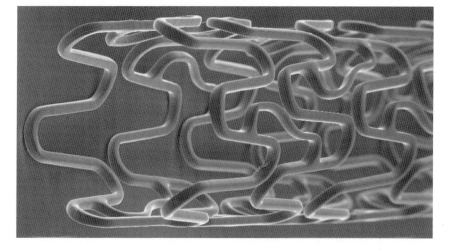

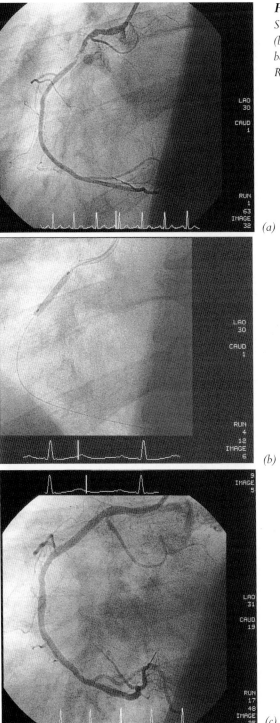

Figure 9.5: *Case 1 (a) Severe proximal RCA stenosis. (b) Appearance of Larus balloon delivery system. (c) Result post-stent deployment.*

(a)

(b)

(c)

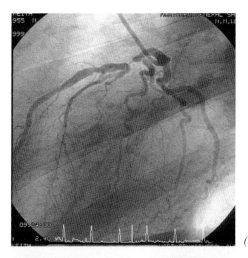

Figure 9.6: Case 2 (a) Extremely severe proximal LAD stenosis. (b) Extensive dissection post-balloon angioplasty.

(a)

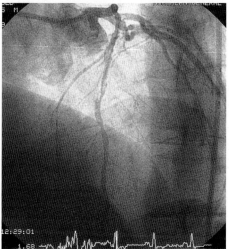

(b)

This dissection required the insertion of four intracoronary stents. Two Coroflex stents were inserted proximally and distally, with two other stents deployed in the mid-portion. The distal Coroflex stent was passed easily through the proximal three stents in order to reach a distal dissection.

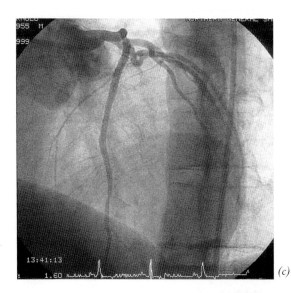

Figure 9.6: Case 2 (c,d)
*Result after stent
implantation.*

(c)

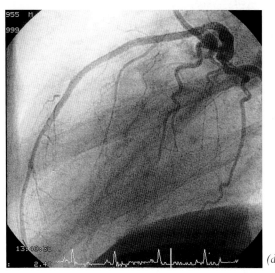

(d)

Clinical trials

There are currently no published trials of the Coroflex stent
*   1998–99: European safety study and 6-month follow up to evaluate
    major adverse cardiac events and restenosis
*   1998–99: International Registry of Coroflex stent implantation

10. THE DURAFLEX™ CORONARY STENT SYSTEM

Avantec Vascular Corporation, San Jose, CA, USA

Guy Leclerc and John Ormiston

Description	The Duraflex™ coronary stent system consists of a laser-cut, stainless steel stent having circumferential rings linked by flexible cross bridges, pre-mounted on a high performance, high pressure, rapid exchange balloon delivery system. This 5 Fr compatible system offers excellent flexibility, high radial strength, low profile, and optimal vessel coverage.

History	• Acute and chronic animal studies conducted that demonstrated results better than or equal to currently marketed stainless steel stents: 2000 • CE mark received: October 2000 • International clinical study: enrolment completed, April 2001 • Japanese clinical study: enrolment underway

Indications for use

De novo lesions
Restenotic lesions
Saphenous vein graft lesions
Suboptimal PTCA
Tortuous anatomy

The Duraflex™ coronary stent technical specifications

Material composition:	316 L stainless steel
Degree of radiopacity (grade):	Moderate
Ferromagnetism:	Non-ferromagnetic (MRI safe)
Metallic surface area expanded:	14% for 3.0 mm diameter
Stent design:	Circumferential rings linked with flexible cross-bridges
Strut dimensions:	0.0050 inch thickness; 0.0042 inch width
Longitudinal flexibility:	High
Percentage shortening on expansion:	Minimal
Degree of recoil (shape memory):	2.2%
Radial force:	High
Currently available diameters:	2.5, 3.0, 3.5, 4.0 mm
Currently available lengths:	8, 14, 18, 25 mm
Other non-coronary types available:	In development

The Duraflex™ stent delivery system

Mechanism of deployment:	Balloon expandable
Minimal recommended guiding catheter:	5 Fr (0.058 inch, 1.47 mm)
Balloon types:	Rapid exchange
Balloon characteristics:	Semi-compliant
Balloon material:	Optimax™
Offered as a bare stent:	No
Protective sheath:	No
Nominal pressure:	9 atm
Rated burst pressure:	16 atm
Delivery profile:	2.5 mm − 0.040 inch (1.02 mm) 3.0 mm − 0.042 inch (1.07 mm) 3.5 mm − 0.043 inch (1.09 mm) 4.0 mm − 0.044 inch (1.12 mm)
Position of radiopaque markers:	Proximal and distal to the stent
Stent retention:	Excellent
Sizing diameter:	Matching target vessel diameter
Recrossability of implanted stents:	Excellent

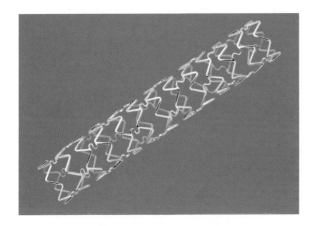

Figure 10.1:
Photograph of the
Duraflex™ stent after
expansion.

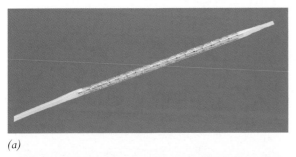

(a)

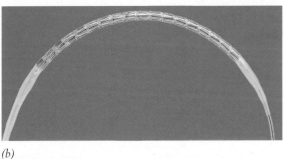

(b)

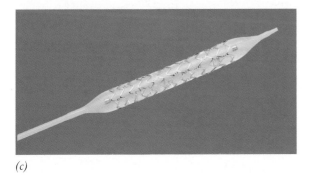

(c)

Figure 10.2:
Photographs of
Duraflex™ stent
delivery system. (a)
Unexpanded system. (b)
The Duraflex stent
system is highly
flexible. (c) Expanded
system (3.0 ×
18 mm).

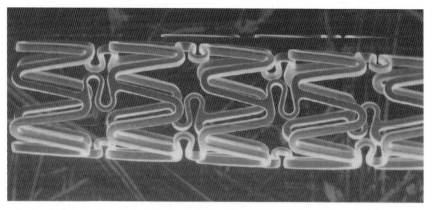

Figure 10.3:
Scanning electron microscope image of the Duraflex™ stent.

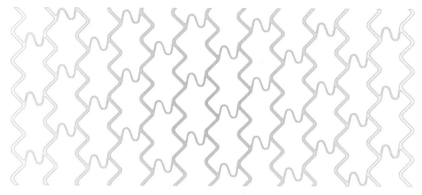

Figure 10.4:
Drawing of Duraflex™ stent pattern. Circumferential rings are linked by flexible cross-bridges. The pattern minimizes the distance between the struts, providing optimal coverage.

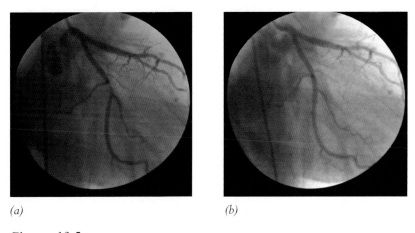

(a)   (b)

Figure 10.5:

(a) A high-grade stenosis in the left circumflex coronary artery. A 3.0 × 14 mm Duraflex™ was implanted by direct stenting through a 5 Fr guiding catheter. The delivery system was inflated to 18 atm. (b) Excellent final result with maintenance of flow in all side branches.

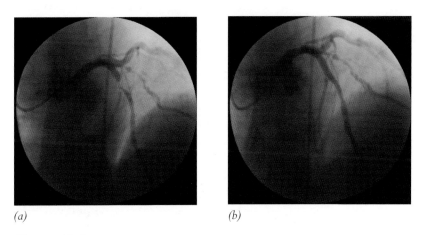

(a)   (b)

Figure 10.6:

(a) A high-grade eccentric stenosis in the left anterior descending coronary artery. A 3.0 × 14 mm Duraflex™ was implanted by direct stenting through a 5 Fr guiding catheter. (b) Post-dilatation of the proximal portion of the stent with a 3.5 × 10 mm balloon optimized the result. Patency of the compromised sidebranch was preserved.

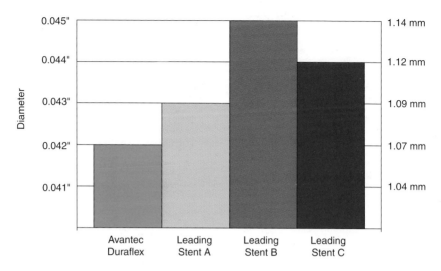

Figure 10.7:

The Duraflex™ has a lower crossing profile than the three leading stent systems (comparison of 3.0 mm stents).

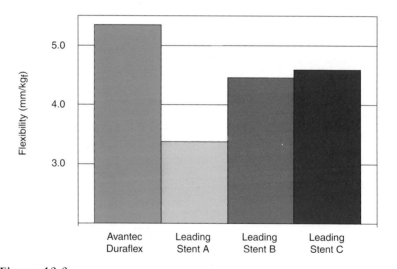

Figure 10.8:

The Duraflex™ stent system is more flexible than the stent systems of the three leading competitors. (Amount stent system bends, mm per kg_f.)

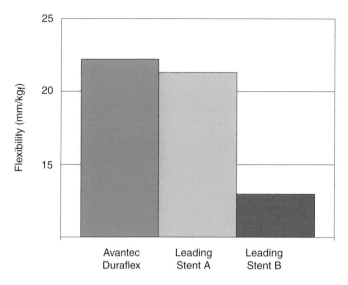

Figure 10.9:

The expanded Duraflex™ stent is more flexible than the leading tubular stents. (Amount expanded stent bends, mm per kgₚ.)

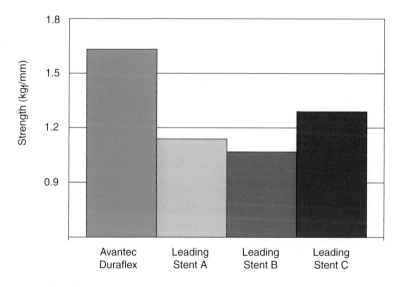

Figure 10.10:

The expanded Duraflex™ stent is stronger than the three leading stents. (Force required to reduce stent diameter in flat plate testing, kgₚ per mm.)

Why I like my stent

The Duraflex™ coronary stent system, the first stent from Avantec, has superior clinical performance as predicted by bench-top testing comparisons with leading competitors. The stent delivery system is highly trackable, with a low stent crossing profile (Figure 10.7) and greater longitudinal flexibility compared with stents of major competitors (Figure 10.8). When expanded, the stent is more flexible than the leading tubular stents (Figure 10.9), allowing for excellent conformability in tortuous anatomy with minimal vessel straightening and minimal arterial distortion at the ends of the stent.

- Although flexibility is high, radial strength is not compromised and is better than major competitor stents (Figure 10.10).
- The unique flexible cross-bridge configuration (Figure 10.4) allows excellent side branch access for bifurcation stenting while retaining scaffolding and coverage properties.
- Radiopacity of this stainless steel stent is optimal in that it allows the stent to be precisely located within the artery without compromise of lumen visibility during coronary angiography.
- The delivery balloon, closely matched to stent length, has high pressure capability and reliable compliance. The excellent stent retention, low crossing profile and pushability (the DriveShaft™ transitional element efficiently transmits push from proximal shaft to distal segment) facilitate direct stenting, when appropriate.
- The low profile allows easy compatibility with contemporary 5 Fr guiding catheters.

Tips and tricks

No special techniques or training required because the system behaves very much like a balloon dilatation catheter. Slow inflation of the balloon ensures excellent concentric expansion of the stent. The low profile, excellent trackability, pushability, and superb stent retention allow for quick and easy direct stenting of appropriately selected lesions.

11. THE EXPRESS CORONARY STENT SYSTEM

Boston Scientific Inc., Natick, MA, USA

Brendon J Pittman

Description	• Balloon expandable stent • Laser cut from a stainless steel tube • Multiple rings connected with multiple links

Design	• Two different elements combined in one single design, offering a balance between flexibility and scaffolding, while addressing a host of other performance attributes.

History	• 2001 CE Marked • Expected FDA approval 2002

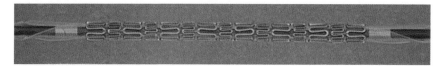

Figure 11.1: *Photo of stent on tube only.*

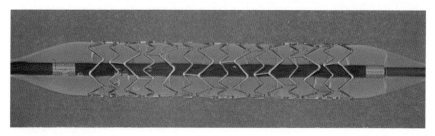

Figure 11.2: *Photo of deployed system.*

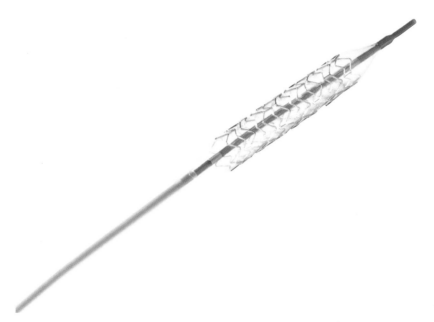

Figure 11.3: *Deployed stent.*

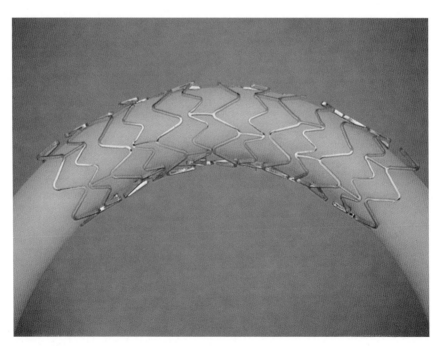

Figure 11.4: *Photo of stent in bend position*

Express coronary stent technical specifications

Material composition:	316 L stainless steel
Degree of radiopacity (grade):	Moderate
Ferromagnetism:	Non-ferromagnetic (MRI safe)
Metallic surface area (metal: artery, expanded):	11–17%
Stent design:	Laser cut from a stainless steel tube in a corrugate ring pattern of Macro and Micro elements
Strut dimensions:	0.0052 inch thick 0.0024/0.0036 inch wide
Longitudinal flexibility:	High
Radial force:	High
Degree of recoil (shape memory):	Minimal
Side branch access:	Excellent
Percentage of shortening on expansion:	< 5% for all sizes
Currently available lengths:	8, 12,16, 20, 24, 28, 32 mm
Currently available diameters:	2.25, 2.5, 2.75, 3.0, 3.5, 4.0, 4.5, 5.0 mm
Recrossibility of implanted stents:	Excellent
Other non-coronary types available:	In development

The Express stent delivery system

Mechanism of deployment:	Balloon expandable
Minimal recommended guiding catheter:	2.25 to 4.0 mm diameters; 5 Fr
Balloon types:	Rapid Exchange and over-the-wire
Balloon characteristics:	High pressure, semi-compliant
Balloon material:	Dynaleap
Offered as a bare stent:	No
Protective sheath:	No
Balloon compliance:	Nominal at 9 atm; + 1/4 size at approx 14 atm
Rated burst pressure of balloon:	2.25–4.0 mm; 18 atm 4.0–5.0 mm; 16 atm
Longitudinal flexibility:	High
Recrossibility of implanted stents:	High
Stent retention:	High
Delivery profile:	2.25–4.0 mm; 2.7 Fr 4.5–5.0 mm; 3.0 Fr

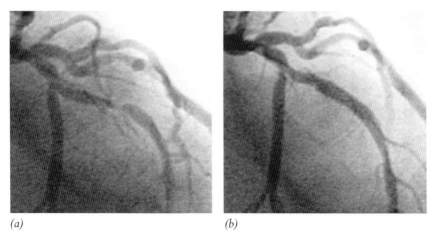

(a)   *(b)*

Figure 11.5: *(a) Pre-procedure; (b) post-procedure.*

12. THE GENIC DYLYN STENT

Blue Medical Devices BV, Helmond, The Netherlands

Henk JM Meens and Ronald AM Horvers

Description   The GENIC® DYLYN® is a DYLYN® coated balloon expandable coronary stent with a helical sinusoidal waveform geometry based on the proven technology of the GENIC®. (For details on the GENIC® stent, see GENIC® specific sections.)

Why I like my stent

The patented DYLYN® coating consists of double amorphous interpenetrating networks, C:H (carbon:hydrogen) and Si:O (silicon:oxygen). DYLYN®'s coating technology and characteristics ensure a direct secure single layer connection to stainless steel. The interpenetrating networks generate a coating with an extremely low surface energy (25–30 mN/m) and a very low surface roughness (0.02 µm Ra) resulting in its strong anti-sticking character. Due to the ultra thin DYLYN® film (<0.5 µm) and the specific network, this coating has an excellent elasticity modulus (<100 Gpa) compared to stainless steel (+200 Gpa), giving it high flexibility. This prevents cracking during expansion of the metal surface, ensuring complete coverage in all phases. The combination of the unique coating characteristics with the geometric flexibility of the GENIC® creates optimal safety and protection features. This combination increases the biocompatibility of the implant, thus decreasing potential restenosis rates. The smooth surface and excellent performance of the coated stent is a suitable one for the application of drug-eluting coating technology.

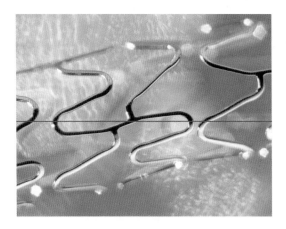

Figure 12.1: *Section of an expanded GENIC® DYLYN® stent.*

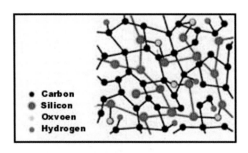

Figure 12.2: *Structure of DYLYN® monocomposite coating.*

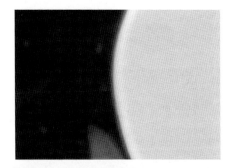

Figure 12.3: *Corner detail of a GENIC® DYLYN® stent strut, showing an homogenate-coated surface with an average thickness of 300 nm. (× 4158).*

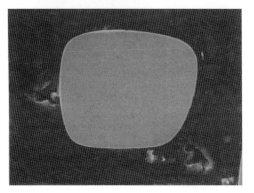

Figure 12.4: *Cross-section of a GENIC® DYLYN® stent strut, showing a homogenate-smooth-coated outside surface, both inside and outside of the strut, with an average thickness of 300 nm. (× 520).*

GENIC® DYLYN® coronary stent family technical specifications

	GENIC® DYLYN®	GENIC® DYLYN® LV	GENIC® DYLYN® SV
Material composition:	316 L medical grade DYLYN® coated	316 L medical grade DYLYN® coated	316 L medical grade DYLYN® coated
Radiopacity:	Moderate	Moderate	Moderate
Ferromagnetism:	Non-ferromagnetic	Non-ferromagnetic	Non-ferromagnetic
MRI:	MRI safe	MRI safe	MRI safe
Metallic surface area			
Expanded:	14% at dia 3.0 mm	14.4% at dia 4.0 mm	14.4% at dia 2.5 mm
Unexpanded:	28%	30%	26%
Metallic cross-sectional area:	0.14 mm^2	0.17 mm^2	0.11 mm^2
Stent design:	Helical sinusoidal waves	Helical sinusoidal waves	Helical sinusoidal waves
Strut design:	Rectangular with rounded edges	Rectangular with rounded edges	Rectangular with rounded edges
Strut dimensions:	0.11–0.12 mm wide	0.10–0.13 mm wide	0.08 × 0.10 mm wide
Strut angles:	N/A	N/A	N/A
Strut thickness:	0.10 mm	0.11 mm	0.09 mm
Mesh angle:	N/A	N/A	N/A
Mesh braid angle:	N/A	N/A	N/A
Profiles			
Bare stent:	N/A	N/A	N/A
Expanded:	2.5–4.0 mm	4.0–5.0 mm	2.0–2.5 mm
Crimped:	<1.0 mm (3.0 × 28)	≤ 1.1 mm (all sizes)	≤ 0.9 mm (all sizes)
Longitudinal flexibility:			
Balloon/stent assy:	Excellent	Excellent	Excellent
Expanded stent:	Excellent	Excellent	Excellent
Shortening (delivery):	N/A	N/A	N/A
Shortening (expansion):	3–4% (3.0 × 18)	4–5% (4.5 × 22)	2–3% (2.5 × 14)
Expansion range:	2.3–4.5 mm	3.7–5.5 mm	1.8–2.8 mm
Recoil:	3–5% (all sizes)	3.5–5.5% (all sizes)	2.5–4.5% (all sizes)
Radial force:	Excellent	Excellent	Excellent
Available diameters:	2.5, 3.0, 3.5, 4.0 mm	4.0, 4.5, 5.0 mm	2.0, 2.5 mm
Available lengths			
Mounted:	10, 14, 18, 22, 28 mm	18, 22, 28 mm	10, 14, 18 mm
Unmounted:	N/A	N/A	N/A
Available sizes:	Full matrix	Full matrix	Full matrix
Recrossability:	Excellent	Excellent	Excellent
Other types:	Under development	Under development	Under development

In vivo biocompatibility

The in vivo biocompatibility of DYLYN® and Diamond-Like stent coating (DLC) was evaluated in a porcine stent model at the Department of Cardiac Research (Professor Ivan de De Scheerder), KUL, Leuven, Belgium. Either DYLYN® coated, DLC top-layer or non-coated stents were randomly implanted in two coronary arteries of 20 pigs. Quantitative coronary analysis, before, immediately after stent implantation, and at 6 weeks, was performed. Morphometry was performed using a computerized morphometric program. Angiographic analysis showed similar baseline selected arteries and post-stenting diameters. At 6 weeks follow-up, there was no significant difference in minimal stent diameter. Histopathology revealed a similar injure score in the three groups. Inflammation was significantly increased in the group of DLC top-layer implanted stents. Thrombus formation was significantly decreased in both coated stent groups. Neointimal hyperplasia was decreased in both coated stent-groups; however, compared to the non-coated stents the difference was not statistically significant. Area stenosis was lower in the DYLYN® coated stent group than in the control group (41 ± 17 vs $54 \pm 15\%$, $P = 0.06$). The results indicate that the double amorphous nanocomposite stent coating (DYLYN®) behaves as a biocompatible stent coating, resulting in a decreased thrombogenicity and decreased neointimal hyperplasia compared to stainless steel. The diamond-like carbon (DLC) film top-layer resulted in an increased inflammatory reaction.

Studies with GENIC® and GENIC® DYLYN®

Ongoing studies

- DIGEST®: multicenter prospective, Benelux registry on the procedural results of direct coronary implantation of the Blue Medical Devices stent.
- DIGESTIVE®: multicenter prospective, longitudinal registry on the procedural results of direct coronary implantation of the Blue Medical Devices stent via 5 Fr guiding catheters.

Planned studies

- Randomized multicenter Trial (460 patients) with 6 months angiographic follow-up starting June 2001.

13. THE GENIC®; GENIC® SV AND GENIC® LV STENT SYSTEMS

Blue Medical Devices B.V., Helmond, The Netherlands

Henk JM Meens and Ronald AM Horvers

Description	The GENIC® is a balloon expandable coronary stent with a helical sinusoidal waveform geometry.

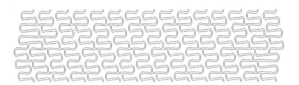

Figure 13.1:
Structure of the GENIC coronary stent.

History	• July–November 1999 development
	• December 1999 completing animal trials
	• December 1999 Development DYLYN®
	• January 2000 CE Mark
	• January 2000 first human implants
	• May 2000 Development SV/LV
	• December 2000 Development drug delivery
	• January 2001 CE Mark SV/LV
	• March 2001 CE Mark DYLYN®

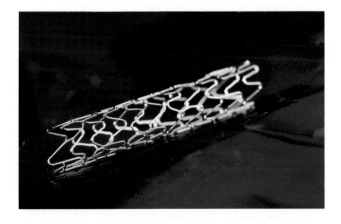

Figure 13.2:
Expanded 18 mm GENIC coronary stent.

GENIC® coronary stent technical specifications

Material composition:	316 L medical grade
Radiopacity:	Moderate
Ferromagnetism:	Non-ferromagnetic
MRI:	MRI safe
Metallic surface area	
expanded:	14% at dia 3.0 mm
unexpanded:	28%
Metallic cross-sectional area:	0.14 mm^2
Stent design:	Helical sinusoidal waves
Strut design:	Rectangular with rounded edges
Strut dimensions:	0.11–0.12 mm wide
Strut thickness:	0.10 mm
Profiles	
expanded:	2.5–4.0 mm
crimped:	< 1.0 mm (3.0 × 28)
Longitudinal flexibility	
Balloon/stent assy:	Excellent
Expanded stent:	Excellent
Shortening (expansion):	3–4% (3.0 × 18)
Expansion range:	2.3–4.5 mm
Recoil:	3–5% (all sizes)
Radial force:	Excellent
Available diameters:	2.5, 3.0, 3.5 and 4.0
Available lengths	
Mounted:	10, 14, 18, 22 and 28
Available sizes:	Full matrix
Recrossability:	Excellent
Other types:	Under development

GENIC® LV coronary stent technical specifications

Material composition:	316 L medical grade
Radiopacity:	Moderate
Ferromagnetism:	Non-ferromagnetic
MRI:	MRI safe
Metallic surface area	
expanded:	14% at dia. 4.0 mm
unexpanded:	30%
Metallic cross-sectional area:	0.17 mm²
Stent design:	Helical sinusoidal waves
Strut design:	Rectangular with rounded edges
Strut dimensions:	0.10–0.13 mm wide
Strut thickness:	0.11 mm
Profiles	
expanded:	4.0–5.0 mm
crimped:	≤ 1.1 mm (all sizes)
Longitudinal flexibility	
Balloon/stent assy:	Excellent
Expanded stent:	Excellent
Shortening (expansion):	4–5% (4.5 × 22)
Expansion range:	3.7–5.5 mm
Recoil:	3.5–5.5% (all sizes)
Radial force:	Excellent
Available diameters:	4.0, 4.5 and 5.0
Available lengths	
Mounted:	18, 22 and 28
Available sizes:	Full matrix
Recrossability:	Excellent
Other types:	Under development

GENIC® SV coronary stent technical specifications

Material composition:	316 L medical grade
Radiopacity:	Moderate
Ferromagnetism:	Non-ferromagnetic
MRI:	MRI safe
Metallic surface area	
expanded:	14% at dia 4.0 mm
unexpanded:	26%
Metallic cross-sectional area:	0.11 mm²
Stent design:	Helical sinusoidal waves
Strut design:	Rectangular with rounded edges
Strut dimensions:	0.08 × 0.10 mm wide
Strut thickness:	0.09 mm
Profiles	
expanded:	2.0–2.5 mm
crimped:	≤ 0.9 mm (all sizes)
Longitudinal flexibility	
Balloon/stent assy:	Excellent
Expanded stent:	Excellent
Shortening (expansion):	2–3% (2.5 × 14)
Expansion range:	1.8–2.8 mm
Recoil:	2.5–4.5% (all sizes)
Radial force:	Excellent
Available diameters:	2.0 and 2.5
Available lengths	
Mounted:	10, 14 and 18
Available sizes:	Full matrix
Recrossability:	Excellent
Other types:	Under development

Tips and tricks for delivery

- The GENIC® coronary stent is premounted on a semi-compliant, high-pressure rapid exchange stent delivery catheter, with optimized pushability and distal flexibility, securing reliable performance.
- The GENIC® coronary stent is positioned between two platinum iridium balloon markers.
- The GENIC® coronary stent delivery system is compatible with a 5 Fr guiding catheter.
- After delivery the GENIC® coronary stent conforms to the natural anatomy of the coronary artery.

Indications for use

- The very flexible GENIC® coronary stent can be applied in a wide range of procedures, from straight stent procedures to procedures in complex tortuous paths and direct stenting.
- The GENIC® coronary stent enables side branch access without decrease of robustness in the design.

Why I like my stent

- The unique geometric design of the GENIC® combines the well-appreciated flexibility of coil stents with the proven robustness of the tubular stents. The superb crimping technology enables direct stenting even through 5 Fr guiding catheters.
- The GENIC® coronary stent is designed to provide optimal flexibility mounted on the stent delivery system.
- Due to this optimal combination, the GENIC® coronary stent and its stent delivery system has an extremely low profile and an excellent crossing performance.
- The helical sinusoidal waveform geometry conforms to the natural dynamic tortuous coronary anatomy and prevents stretching of the vessel. This excellent flexibility allows placement in very dynamic coronary anatomy with less stress on the coronary vessel wall preventing restenosis at the extremities.

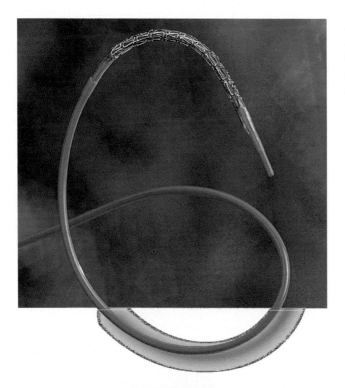

Figure 13.3:
Flexibility of the GENIC coronary stent delivery system.

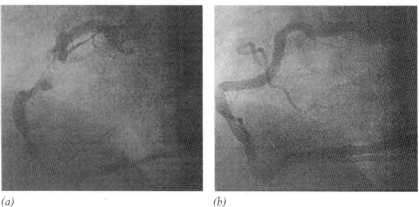

(a)   (b)

Figure 13.4: *(a) Complete stenosis in tortuous proximal right coronary artery; (b) after GENIC stent implantation. This shows the excellent conformability to the vessel wall of the expanded stent.*

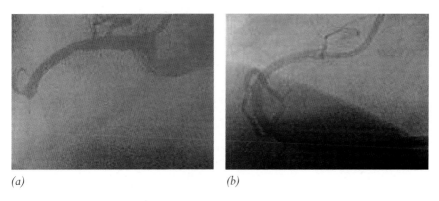

(a)   *(b)*

Figure 13.5: *(a) Total occlusion of proximal right coronary artery; (b) after recanalization and GENIC stent implantation.*

Delivery device of GENIC®	
Mechanism of deployment:	Balloon expandable
Minimal internal guiding catheter:	0.056 inch
Maximal guidewire diameter:	0.014 inch
System:	Rapid exchange
Design:	Hypo tube
Proximal shaft:	2.1 Fr
Distal shaft:	2.6 Fr
Number of markers:	2
Type of markers:	Platinum iridium
Position of markers:	Proximal and distal balloon
Position stent:	Between balloon markers
Balloon material:	Acrylon® (thermoplastic elastomer)
Compliance:	Semi-compliant, high-pressure
Nominal:	6 atm
Rated burst pressure:	16 atm (> 4.0 mm: 14 atm.)
GENIC® is a registered trademark of Blue Medical Devices	

14. THE GENIUS CORONARY STENT

EuroCor GmbH, Bonn, Germany

Thomas A Ischinger and Michael Orlowski

Description
- Balloon expandable tubular stent
- Multicellular – modular ring design
- Alternating connections with multiple links
- Sheathless and premounted stent system
- Available in lengths of 8, 11, 15, 19, 23, 27 mm and diameters of 2.5–4.0 mm

History
- April 1999 – international market release
- CE mark approval received
- Multi centre registry study finished
- October 1999 randomized trial with 250 patients started
- July 1999 hemocompatibility test report finished
- October 1999 registry study for Japan started
- Multicenter registry study 100 patients, Israel finished, March 2000 long term Genius stent implantation result, 11% restenosis rate
- Genius complex lesion stenting study, Lesion B2 and C, finished, January 2001 by Reifart et al.
- Genius immediate and long term results after Genius stent implantation, Ischinger et al.

Genius stent technical specifications

Material composition:	316L stainless steel
Degree of radiopacity (grade):	Good
Ferromagnetism:	Non-ferromagnetic (MRI safe)
Metal surface area (metal: artery, expanded):	17% average
Stent design:	Multicellular-modular ring design Alternating connections with multiple links
Strut design:	Tubular, smooth rounded
Strut dimensions:	0.004 inch (0.11 mm) thick
Profile: non-expanded (uncrimped):	1.6 mm (0.06 inch)
expanded:	up to 4.5 mm
on the balloon:	0.038 inch
Longitudinal flexibility:	High
Percentage shortening on delivery:	None
Percentage shortening on expansion:	<3%
Expansion range:	2.5–4.0 mm
Degree of recoil (shape memory):	<2%
Radial force (to collapse):	High, excellent
Currently available diameters:	2.5, 2.75, 3.0, 3.5 and 4.0 mm
Currently available lengths:	
Mounted	9, 11, 15, 19, 23, 27 mm
unmounted	9, 11, 15, 19, 23, 27 mm
Currently available sizes:	2.5–4 mm
Re-crossability of implanted stent:	Excellent
Other non-coronary types:	No

Genius coronary stent delivery system

Mechanism of deployment:	Balloon expandable
Mechanism of expanding:	Balloon expandable
Minimum internal diameter of guiding catheter:	0.064 inch (1.6 mm) 5 Fr
Monorail system:	Yes
Balloon characteristics:	Semi-compliant, moderately
Balloon material:	Polyamide
Guidewire lumen:	0.014 inch (0.36 mm)
Minimum recommended guide:	5 Fr
Premounted on delivery cath:	Yes
Premounted on high pressure B:	Yes
Protected sheath cover:	No
Offered as a bare stent:	Yes
Position of radio-opaque markers:	Proximal and distal stent ends
Rated burst pressure of balloon:	16 atm for 2.5–3.5 mm 14 atm for 4.0 mm
Delivery balloon compliance:	Semi-compliant, moderately
Delivery profile (crossing profile):	0.038–0.040 inch
Longitudinal flexibility:	Excellent
Recommended deployment pressure:	Nominal at 9 atm
Further balloon expansion recommended:	At physician's discretion
Balloon dilatation and stent sizing:	Equal to artery or up to 10%
Recrossability of implanted stent:	Excellent
Sizing diameter:	2.5–4.5 mm

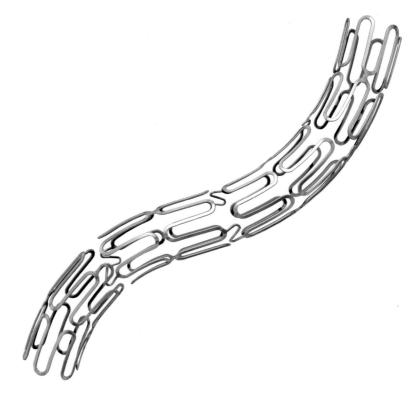

Figure 14.1: Genius coronary stent.

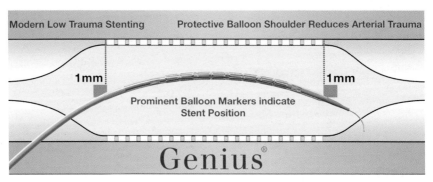

Figure 14.2: Genius low trauma stenting.

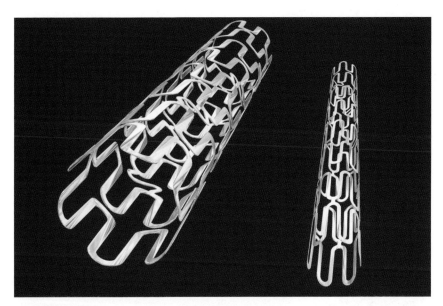

Figure 14.3: Genius stent expanded.

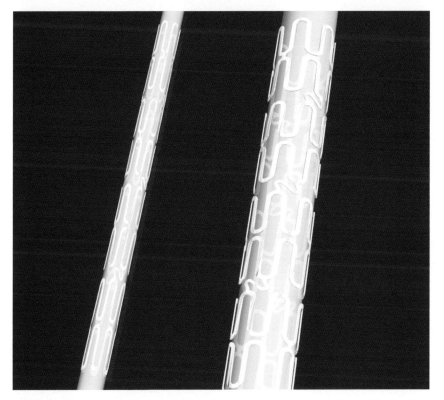

Figure 14.4: Genius stent mounted.

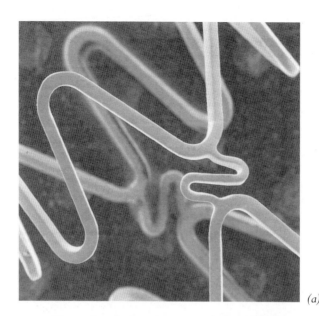

Figure 14.5: *(a) Genius stent expanded; (b) Genius stent expanded, 300 µm.*

(a)

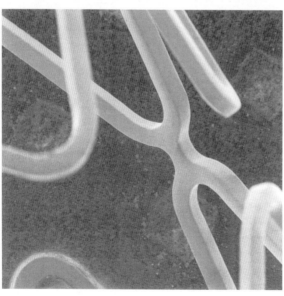

(b)

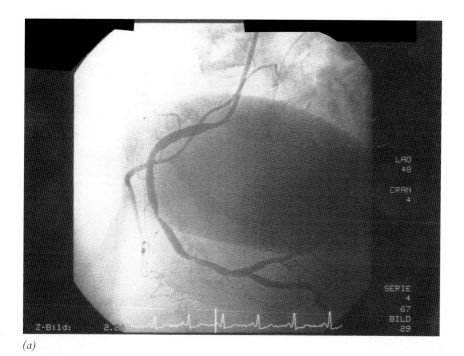

(a)

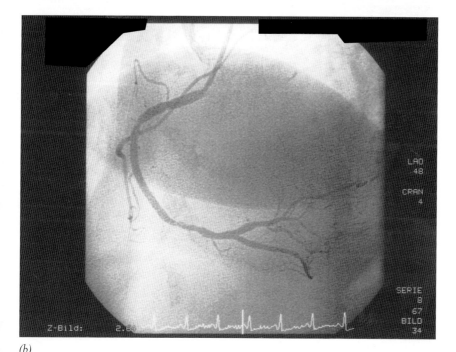

(b)

Figure 14.6: *Genius direct stenting (a) before; (b) after.*

Current indications for clinical use

• Native coronary arteries, de novo and restenotic lesions

Why I like my stent

• Superb flexibility, ideal for tortuous anatomy
• Very low crossing profile, ideal for tight lesions and narrow and distal arteries
• Stent opens homogeneously
• Overexpansion in order to make up for recoil is never necessary thus making very atraumatic placements possible.
• Specially treated metal and mesh design result in optimal performance profile: perfect compliance with vessel wall stability (optimal radial strength, no recoil) and flexibility.
• Balloon ends are soft and comply very well with the often healthy segment of the vessel wall at the ends of the stent, to avoid unnecessary injury.
• Genius opens at relatively low pressures, another safety and minimize trauma feature
• Excellent radial force makes the stent good for hard calcified lesions.
• The stent can be easily advanced through stents due to its smooth and rounded strut features.
• Side branch access is well preserved by the particular mesh design.
• Very good for bifurcation stenting.
• Good visualization with two gold markers.
• Excellent scaffolding.

Studies in which the stent is involved

• Stent registry study 100 patients, finished (European).
• Haemocompatibility study, finished (University of Homburg).
• Randomized multicentre trial (250 patients); started October 1999 with angiographic follow-up at 6 months, finished.
• Stent registry study 100 patients for Japan approval; 6 months follow-up, started July 2001
• Three different antiproliferative agents will be tested
• Genius drug coating during stent trials: 400 patients

15. THE IGAKI-TAMAI® STENT

Igaki Medical Planning, Kyoto, Japan

Hideo Tamai and Takafumi Tsuji

Description	The Igaki-Tamai® Stent is the first biodegradable stent to be implanted in humans. It is made of PLLA (poly-L-lactic acid) mono-polymer and has a zigzag helical coil design. The stent is a pre-mounted balloon-expandable device, which also has a self-expanding capacity, and carries two radiopaque markers. The Igaki-Tamai® polymer stent biodegrades in 1–1.5 years.

History	1994	Development of knitted design polymer stent
	1995	Early animal trials
	1996	First implant in porcine coronary arteries with knitted design PLLA stent
	1997	Development of zigzag helical coil design PLLA stent
	April 1998	Implant in porcine coronary arteries with zigzag helical coil design PLLA stent
	September 1998	First human implant in Japan
	September 1999	First human implant in Europe
	September 2000	Development of new delivery system without protective sheath
	Future	Development of drug delivery system, with PLLA stent

Igaki-Tamai® Stent technical specifications

Material composition:	PLLA(poly-L-lactic acid) medical grade
Degree of radiopacity (grade):	Moderate
Polymer surface area (polymer:artery expanded):	24% at 3.0 mm diameter
Ferromagnetism:	Non-ferromagnetic (MRI safe)
Polymer cross-sectional area:	0.013 inch² (0.32 mm²)
Stent design:	Zigzag helical coil
Longitudinal flexibility:	High
Radiopaque markers:	Proximal and distal edges
Strut thickness:	0.007 inch (0.17 mm)
Currently available length:	12 mm
Other non-coronary types:	No
Expansion range:	3.0–4.5 mm
Percentage shortening on expansion:	< 0.8% at 4.0 mm diameter
Currently available diameters:	3.0, 3.5, 4.0 mm

Igaki-Tamai® Stent delivery system previous

Mechanism of deployment:	Balloon expandable
Minimal internal diameter of guiding catheter:	0.086 inch (2.18 mm), 8 Fr
Premounted on delivery catheter:	Yes
Protective sheath:	Yes
Further dilatation recommended:	At physician's discretion
Recommended deployment pressure:	Nominal
Available bare (unmounted):	No

Igaki-Tamai® Stent delivery system introduced September 2000

Mechanism of deployment:	Balloon
Premounted on delivery catheter:	Yes
Protective sheath:	No
Balloon types:	Rapid exchange & over the wire
Longitudinal flexibility	High

New delivery system

Igaki-Tamai® Stent is a self-expanding stent. In the previous version a protective sheath was used to retain the stent on the delivery system. With the new stent delivery system, the Igaki-Tamai® Stent can be implanted by balloon inflation without sheath. In other words, the implantation of the Igaki-Tamai® Stent can be performed in the same way as any other balloon expandable stents. The Igaki Tamai® Stent is held in the holding system shaped on the balloon. With the balloon inflated, the holding system opens and the stent is released and expanded against the vessel wall. After implantation, the Igaki-Tamai® Stent further expands gradually in the coronary artery.

Indications for clinical use

- De novo lesions
- Restenotic lesions
- Acute closure and bailout situations
- Suboptimal PTCA result
- Acute MI
- Vessels > 2.5 mm
- Lesions with side branch
- Lesions with tortuous anatomy

Clinical data

In hospital results:
In Japan, 63 lesions in 50 patients were treated with the Igaki-Tamai® Stent
Lesion type (AHA/ACC): Type B1 25%, Type B2 57%, Type C 11%
Lesion length: 13.5 ± 5.7 mm
Reference vessel diameter: 2.95 ± 0.46 mm
Angiographic success: 63/63 (100%)
Clinical success: 49/50 (98%)
Subacute stent thrombosis (SAT) with Q-MI: 1/50 (2%)
No death
No emergent bypass surgery

Follow-up results:
Clinical follow-up at 6 months in 50 patients (63 lesions)
Angiographic follow-up at 6 months in 49 patients (60 lesions)
No death
No bypass surgery
Repeat PTCA: 6/50 (12%)
Restenosis (%DS>50%): 11/60 (18%)

QCA results:

	Pre	Post	6 months
MLD (mm)	0.91 ± 0.39	2.68 ± 0.43	1.76 ± 0.74
%DS (%)	69 ± 13	12 ± 8	38 ± 22

Why I like my stent

Although metallic stents are effective in preventing acute occlusion and late restenosis following coronary angioplasty, metallic stents remaining in place are obstacles to additional treatments (e.g., repeat angioplasty and bypass surgery). Acute closure and restenosis commonly occur within 3–6 months following coronary intervention, and rarely thereafter. Therefore the clinical need for stent scaffolding is reduced after 6–9 months. Considering the short-term need, stents made of biodegradable materials may be an ideal alternative. A biodegradable stent may also be useful for the local administration of pharmaceutical agents directly to the site of PTCA to prevent late restenosis. The Igaki-Tamai® stent is a flexible biodegradable and self-expanding stent pre-mounted on a delivery balloon with a protective sheath. The stent gradually expands after implantation and loses the strength beyond 6 months and biodegrades completely after 1–1.5 years. The stent can also be used as a vehicle for local drug therapy. These new functions of stents may improve the long-term efficacy of stents in the treatment of coronary heart disease.

References

1. Zidar J, Lincoff A, Stack R. Biodegradable stents. In: Topol EJ, ed. *Textbook of Interventional Cardiology*, 2nd ed., Philadelphia: WB Saunders, 1994: 787–802.

2. Van der Giessen WJ, Lincoff AM, Schwartz RS *et al*. Marked inflammatory sequelae to implantation of biodegradable and nonbiodegradable polymers in porcine coronary artery. *Circulation* 1996;**94**:1690–7.

3. Lincoff AM, Furst JG, Ellis SG, Tuch RJ, Topol EJ. Sustained local delivery of dexamethasone by a novel intravascular eluting stent to prevent restenosis in the porcine coronary injury model. *J Am Coll Cardiol* 1997;**29**:808–16.

4. Yamawaki T, Shimokawa H, Kozai *et al*. Intramural delivery of a specific tyrosine kinase inhibitor with biodegradable stent suppresses the restenotic changes of the coronary artery in pigs in vivo. *J Am Coll Cardiol* 1998;**32**:780–6.

5. Tamai H, Igaki K, Kyo E, *et al*. Initial and 6-month results of biodegradable poly-L-lactic acid coronary stents in humans. *Circulation* 2000;**102**:399–404.

16. THE JOSTENT® CORONARY STENT RANGE

JOMED AB, Helsingborg, Sweden

Nicolaus Reifart

JOSTENT® Flex

General description

The JOSTENT® Flex is specially designed for complex lesion morphology. The JOSTENT® Flex combines flexibility through spiral links with high radial strength. Thus it combines the favourable properties of a coil stent (flexibility, sidebranch access) with the strength and integrity of a slotted tube stent. This new design provides increased individual cell area and further options that allow implantation in vessels up to 5 mm in diameter.

The JOSTENT® Flex is laser cut from a stainless steel tube and requires no weld points. The stent is then polished leaving a clean surface area with rounded struts. The JOSTENT® Flex is also available pre-mounted on a high performance delivery catheter with a semi-compliant balloon and an extremely low profile of less than 1.1mm.

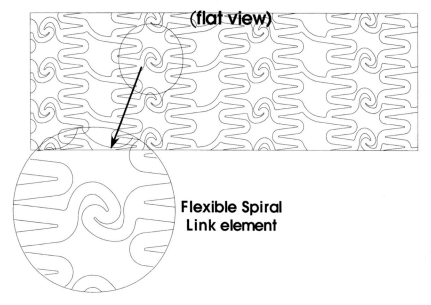

Figure 16.1: *Design JOSTENT® Flex.*

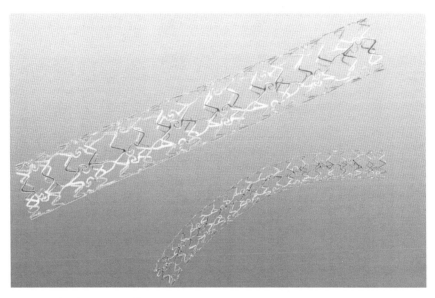

Figure 16.2: *JOSTENT® Flex.*

JOSTENT® Flex technical specifications

Material composition:	316L stainless steel
Degree of radiopacity (grade):	Moderate
Ferromagnetism:	Non-ferromagnetic (MRI safe)
Metallic surface area (metal: artery, expanded):	14–19%
Degree of recoil (shape memory):	<3%
Strut design:	Rounded edges
Strut thickness:	0.0035 inch (0.09 mm)
Delivery profile (crossing profile):	0.04 inch (1 mm)
Longitudinal flexibility:	High
Percentage shortening upon expansion:	<3% at 3.5 mm
Currently available lengths:	9, 12, 16, 19, 26 and 32 mm
Currently available diameters:	2.0–3.25 mm (small vessel version)
	3.0–5.0 mm (standard version)

JOMED PREMOUNTED SYSTEMS

General description	The JOSTENT® Flex Stent is available as bare stent and premounted versions. JOMED is offering the JOSTENT® Flex on two different delivery systems, which are based on different shaft constructions. The JOSTENT® Flex Supreme System has a stiffening wire construction whereas the JOSTENT® FlexMaster is based on a stainless steel shaft construction. Both systems have low crimped profiles and stent security and expansion is supported by a special balloon folding design, the K-folding: a combination of a distal four fold and a proximal un-uniform fold.
	The Plus 1 design allows 1 mm balloon overhang on each side of the stent. The stent is mounted directly onto the markers.

JOSTENT® Flex Supreme System

Mechanism of deployment:	Balloon expandable
Minimal ID of guiding catheter:	0.064 inch (1.63 mm), 6 Fr
Premounted on delivery system:	JOSTENT Flex on semi-compliant balloon
Protective sheath:	No
Position of radiopaque markers:	2 markers, stent is crimped onto markers
Recrossability of implanted stents:	Excellent
Available balloon diameters:	2.5–4.0 mm
Available stent length (premounted):	9, 12, 16, 19, 26 mm
Available bare:	Yes
Coating: available	Also with JOMED Heparin Coating

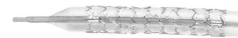

Figure 16.3: JOSTENT® Flex Supreme System.

JOSTENT® FlexMaster

Mechanism of deployment:	Balloon expandable
Minimal ID of guiding catheter:	0.058 inch, 5 Fr
Premounted on delivery system:	JOSTENT® Flex on a semi-compliant balloon, stainless steel shaft construction
Protective sheath:	No
HYDREX coating system:	Hydrophilic coated tip, JET Coating on shaft and guidewire lumen
Position of radiopaque markers:	2 markers, stent is crimped onto markers
Recrossability of implanted stents:	Excellent
Available balloon diameters:	2.5–4.0 mm
Available stent length (premounted):	9, 12, 16, 19, 26 mm
Available bare:	Yes
Coating:	Also with JOMED heparin coating available

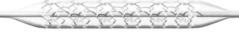

Figure 16.4: JOSTENT® FlexMaster.

JOSTENT® Sidebranch

General description

The JOSTENT® Sidebranch is the first stent specifically developed for sidebranch applications and incorporates larger cells that minimize the risk of sidebranch occlusion and can be expanded up to 6.0 mm in diameter to allow access for further PTCA and stenting of sidebranches.

The JOSTENT® Sidebranch is a combination of JOSTENT® Flex and JOSTENT® Plus. The proximal and distal portions of the stent are based on the Plus design, ensuring high radial strength and flexibility, whereas the mid-portion utilizes the Spiral Links of the JOSTENT® Flex to maximize access to sidebranches. The stent is available in two lengths, 18 and 26 mm.

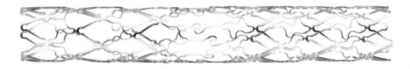

Figure 16.5: JOSTENT® Sidebranch.

JOSTENT® Sidebranch technical specifications

Material composition:	316L stainless steel
Degree of radiopacity (grade):	Moderate
Ferromagnetism:	Non-ferromagnetic (MRI safe)
Metallic surface area (metal: artery, expanded):	14–19%
Degree of recoil (shape memory):	<5%
Strut design:	Rounded edges
Strut thickness:	0.0051 inch (0.13 mm)
Delivery profile (crossing profile):	0.04 inch (1 mm) balloon dependant
Longitudinal flexibility:	High
Percentage shortening upon expansion:	<3% at 3 mm
Currently available lengths:	18 and 26 mm
Currently available diameters:	3.0–6.0 mm

THE JOSTENT® CORONARY STENT RANGE

JOSTENT® Bifurcation

General description	The unique JOSTENT® Bifurcation has been designed for treating lesions in or at bifurcations. It is a combination of the JOSTENT® Flex and JOSTENT® Plus.

The distal portion of the stent is based on the JOSTENT® Plus design, ensuring high radial strength, whereas the proximal portion of the stent utilizes the Spiral Links of the JOSTENT® Flex to maximize access to bifurcations.

The larger cells can be expanded up to 6.0 mm in diameter to allow further stent placement in the bifurcated vessels, allowing the placement of a second stent through the struts of the first stent.

The JOSTENT® Bifurcation is available in two lengths, 16 and 28 mm.

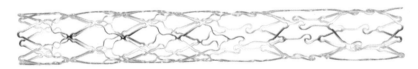

Figure 16.6: JOSTENT® Bifurcation.

JOSTENT® Bifurcation technical specifications

Material composition:	316L stainless steel
Degree of radiopacity (grade):	Moderate
Ferromagnetism:	Non-ferromagnetic (MRI safe)
Metallic surface area (metal: artery, expanded):	14–19%
Degree of recoil (shape memory):	<5%
Strut design:	Rounded edges
Strut thickness:	0.0051 inch (0.13 mm)
Crimped profile:	0.04 inch (1 mm) balloon dependant
Longitudinal flexibility:	High
Percentage shortening upon expansion:	<3% at 3 mm
Currently available lengths:	16 and 28 mm
Currently available diameters:	3.0–6.0 mm

129

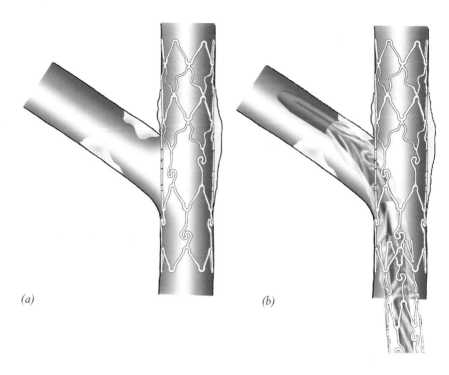

(a)

(b)

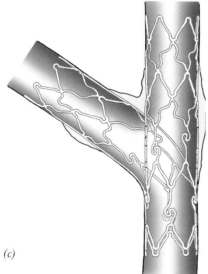

Figure 16.7: *(a) First stent is inserted and expanded. (b) Second stent is introduced. (c) Expansion of second stent – final result.*

(c)

JOSTENT® Coronary Stent Graft

Description   JOMED has developed a unique stent technology which represents a new era in coronary stenting. The JOSTENT® Coronary Stent Graft combines a flexible stent with a layer of expandable PTFE graft material designed for successful management of acute cardiac situations.

The JOSTENT® Coronary Stent Graft combines all the properties of a graft and a coronary stent, yet it is as flexible as most conventional stents. The JOSTENT® Coronary Stent Graft has been constructed by using a unique sandwich technique, whereby an ultrathin layer of expandable PTFE is placed between two stents, welded at its ends.

This design provides high radial strength and longitudinal flexibility and the device can be crimped down to a low profile, very close to standard bare stents (6Fr compatible). The unique construction allows the JOSTENT® Coronary Stent Graft to effectively seal off the vessel wall. It can be safely implanted and is beneficial or even life-saving in coronary dissections, perforations, aneurysms and bypass graft lesions.

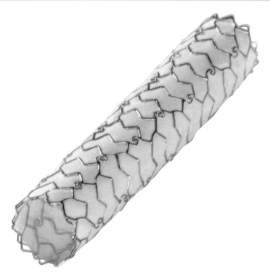

Figure 16.8: JOSTENT® Coronary Stent Graft.

JOSTENT® Coronary Stent Graft technical specifications

Material composition:	316L stainless steel, PTFE
Degree of radiopacity (grade):	Moderate
Ferromagnetism:	Non-ferromagnetic (MRI safe)
Degree of recoil (shape memory):	<5%
Strut design:	Rounded edges
Wall thickness:	0.012 inch (0.30 mm)
Delivery profile (crossing profile):	0.064 inch (1.6 mm)
Longitudinal flexibility:	Good
Percentage shortening upon expansion:	<3% at 3.5 mm
Currently available lengths:	Stent graft length: 9, 12, 16, 19 and 26 mm
Currently available diameters:	2.5 to 5.0 mm
Other non-coronary types:	Vascular, iliac

Tips and tricks for delivery (JOSTENT® Coronary Stent Graft)

- For optimal expansion use inflation pressures of min. 14–16 atm.
- Use IVUS to ensure optimal deployment.

JOSTENT® CORONARY STENT GRAFT SUPREME SYSTEM

Description   JOMED has made the JOSTENT® Coronary Stent Graft available on a delivery system called the Supreme System. This combines a covered stent with a state-of-the-art delivery system.

The JOSTENT® Coronary Stent Graft combines a flexible stent with a layer of expandable PTFE graft material designed for successful management of acute cardiac situations.

The JOSTENT® Coronary Stent Graft possesses all the properties of a graft and a coronary stent, yet it is as flexible as most conventional stents. The JOSTENT® Coronary Stent Graft has been constructed by using a unique sandwich technique, whereby an ultrathin layer of expandable PTFE is placed between two stents, welded at its ends. This design provides high radial strength and longitudinal flexibility. The unique construction allows the JOSTENT® Coronary Stent Graft to seal off the vessel wall effectively. It can be safely implanted and is beneficial or even life-saving in coronary dissections, perforations, aneurysms, fistulas and saphenous bypass graft lesions.

The JOMED Supreme delivery system consists of a low profile, supremely trackable and durable semi-compliant balloon with two markers. The balloon has the "Plus One" design which is a unique design for optimal stent placement and minimal stent edge dissections.

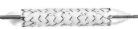

Figure 16.9: JOSTENT® Coronary Stent Graft Supreme System.

JOMED Coronary Stent Graft Supreme System technical specifications

Material composition:	Stainless steel 316 L PTFE Polytetrafluoroethylene
Wall thickness:	0.3 mm
Expansion range:	2.5–5.0 mm
Balloon material:	Semi-compliant
Shaft size:	2.8 Fr
Premounted profile:	≤ 1.6 mm (0.063 inch)
Expansion pressure:	Min. 14 bar
Rated burst pressure:	16 bar
Average burst pressure:	≥ 22 bar
Minimum guiding catheter:	I.D. 0.068 inch
Recommended guidewire:	0.014 inch

Tips and tricks for delivery of the JOSTENT® Coronary Stent Graft

• For optimal expansion use inflation pressures of min. 14–16 bar
• Use IVUS to ensure optimal deployment

CLINICAL EXPERIENCE

JOSTENT® CORONARY STENT GRAFT

Richard R Heuser, Alejandro Lopez, Nicolaus Reifart, Hans Stoerger

Phoenix Heart Center, Phoenix, Arizona, USA; Red Cross Hospital, Frankfurt, Germany

83 JOSTENT® Coronary Stent Graft stents were implanted in 76 patients aged 60.5±10.3 years. The vessels included: SVG (n = 24), RCA (n = 26), LAD (n = 20), and LCX (n = 6). Indications included aneurysm (n = 22), friable SVG (n = 15), thrombotic plaque (n = 7), perforation (n = 4), de novo (n = 20), and restenosis (n = 8 with six having multiple in-stent restenosis). Patients were treated with ASA 300 mg and Ticlopidine 2 × 250 mg (3 weeks). Angiographic success was 97% (74/76) and all four perforations were sealed successfully. A 6Fr guiding catheter was used 33% (25/76). Maximum balloon size was 3.7±0.7 mm with a maximum pressure of 12–24 bar. Pre-procedure stenosis was 81.5±15.4% and post-procedure stenosis was 7.6±18.1%. Complications included one subacute thrombosis after 7 hours. Six month angiographic follow-up was available in six patients and revealed restenosis in 33% (1 with diffuse 60% narrowing and one with focal restenosis at the stent ends).

Conclusions

The PTFE covered JOSTENT® is easy to insert in larger coronary arteries and SVGs and can be used to cover aneurysms, vessel ruptures, and perforations, or as treatment for focal repetitive restenosis. Further investigations are warranted to evaluate the 6 month binary restenosis rate and target revascularization rate.

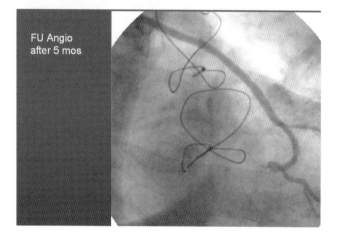

Figure 16.10

Original Studies

Membrane-covered stents: a new treatment strategy for saphenous vein graft lesions

Stephen Baldus, Ralf Köster, Jacobus Reimers, Jan Kähler, Thomas Meinertz and Christian W Hamm

The restenosis rate after stenting of lesions in aortocoronary venous bypass grafts still has to be considered unsatisfactorily high. We investigated a new stent design characterized by an expandable polytetrafluorethylene (PTFE) membrane in between two layers of struts. Five consecutive male patients (age 70 ± 6 years) were followed prospectively who presented with at least two de novo lesions in different grafts 13 ± 3 years after bypass surgery. A total of 11 lesions were treated located in grafts anastomosed to the circumflex ($n = 3$), to the LAD ($n = 7$), and to the right coronary artery

($n = 1$). Within the same procedure, every patient received membrane-covered stents ($n = 6$) and conventional stents ($n = 5$) in either of their lesions. All patients underwent successful interventions. The minimal luminal diameter increased from 1.0 ± 0.5 to 2.9 ± 0.6 mm in lesions treated by the membrane-covered stents and from 0.8 ± 0.4 to 2.4 ± 0.7 mm in the lesions treated by conventional stents. During follow-up, four out of five patients required angioplasty for in-stent restensosis of lesions covered by a conventional stent, whereas no patient underwent revascularization for a lesion treated by a membrane-covered device. The mean minimal luminal diameter of lesions covered by a conventional stent decreased by 42% to 1.4 ± 0.6 mm; the mean minimal luminal diameter of the lesions treated by a stent graft declined by 9% to 2.8 ± 0.6 mm ($P < 0.05$). This series of intraindividual comparisons suggests the membrane-covered stents may have the power to reduce in-stent restenosis in obstructed aortocoronary venous bypass grafts.

References

1. Gerckens U, Müller R, Cattelaens N, Herchenbach M, Grube E. The new coronary stent graft JOSTENT® first clinical experience [abstract]. *J Am Coll Cardiol* 1998;**31**.

2. Elsner E, Auch-Schwelk W, Walter DH, Schachinger V, Zeiher AM. Evolving coronary application of stent grafts containing a polytetrafluorethylen-membrane [abstract]. *Eur Heart J* 1998;**19**.

3. Lopez A, Heuser RH, Störger H, Reifart N. Coronary artery application of an endoluminal polytetrafluorethylene stent graft: two center experience with the Jomed JOSTENT®. *AHA November 1998*.

4. Morice M-C, Louvard Y, Maillard L, Guemonprez JL, Kahlife K, Druelles P, Chevalier B, Hirsch JL, Wittenberg O, Boccara A, Valeix B, Cribier A, Nicolle C. French registry of coronary stent grafts: acute and mid-term results. *AHA November 1998*.

5. Heuser RR, Woodfield S, Lopez A. Obliteration of a coronary artery aneurysm with a PTFE covered stent: the endoluminal graft for coronary disease revisited. *Cathet Cardiovasc Diag* 1998;**7**.

6. Elsner M, Zeiher AM. Perforation and rupture of coronary arteries. *Herz* 1998;**23**:311–318.

7. Gerckens U, Müller R, Cattelaens N, Büllesfeld L, Herchenbach M, Grube E. First clinical experiences with a covered stent: the JOSTENT® coronary stent graft. *Int J Cardiovasc Intervent* 1998;**1**:68–74.

8. von Birgelen C, Haude M, Liu F, Ge J, Görge G, Welge D, Wieneke H, Baumgart D, Opherk D, Erbel R. Treatment of coronary

pseudoaneurysm by stent–graft implantation. *Deutsche Medizinische Wochenschrift* 1998;**123**:418–422.

9. Lotze U, Ferrari M, Dannberg G, Kühnert H, Figulla HR. Unexpanded, irretrievable stent in the proximal right coronary artery: successful management with stent-graft implantation. *Cathet Cardiovasc Intervent* 1999;**46**:344–349.

10. Baldus S, Zeiher A, Reimers J, Elsner M, Schaps KP, Gerckens U, Grube E, Büllesfeld L, Hamm CW. Reduction of restenosis in venous bypass graft lesions after implantation of a covered graft stent. *ACCIS'99*.

11. Gerckens U, Müller R, Cattelaens N, Rowold S, Grube E. Coronary stent graft JOSTENT® versus conventional stent design in complex coronary lesions. *ACCIS'99*.

12. De Gregorio J, Corvaja N, Adamian M, Kobayashi N, Moussa I, Reimers B, Di Francesco L, Vaghetti M, Finci L, Kobayashi Y, Albiero R, Di Mario C, Colombo A. Experience with the PTFE covered stent in percutaneous coronary interventional procedures: indications and outcome. *ACCIS'99*.

13. Morice M-C, Kumar R, Levèvre T, Loubeyre C, Morelle J-F, Traisnel G, Commeau P, Labrunie P, Berland J, Royer T, Henry M. The French registry of coronary stent grafts: acute and term results. *ACCIS'99*.

14. Elsner M, Britten M, Auch-Schwelk W, Walter DH, Schächinger V, Zeiher AM. Distribution of neointimal proliferation in human coronary arteries treated with polytetrafluorethylene stent-grafts. *ACCIS'99*.

15. Elsner M, Auch-Schwelk W, Walter DH, Schächinger V, Zeiher AM. Stent-grafts containing a polytetrafluorethylene-membrane: emerging indications for implantation into human coronary arteries. *ACCIS'99*.

16. Albiero R, Nishida T, Corvaja N, et al. Left internal mammary artery graft perforation repair using polytetrafluoroethylene-covered stents. *Cathet Cardiovasc Intervent* 2000;**51**:78–82.

17. Briguori C, Nishida T, Anzuini A, et al. Emergency polytetrafluoroethylene-covered stent implantation to treat coronary ruptures. *Circulation* 2000;**102**:3028–31.

18. Roongsritong C, Laothavorn P, Sa-nguanwong S. Stent grafting for coronary arteriovenous fistula with adjacent atherosclerotic plaque in a patient with myocardial infarction. *J Invasive Cardiol* 2000;**12**:283–5.

19. Baldus S, Koster R Elsner M, et al. Treatment of aortocoronary vein graft lesions with membrane-covered stents: a multicenter surveillance trial. *Circulation* 2000;**102**:2024–7.

20. Briguori C, De Gregorio J, Nishida T, et al. Polytetrafluoroethylene-covered stent for the treatment of narrowings in aorticoronary saphenous vein grafts. *Am J Cardiol* 2000;**86**:343–6.

21. Baldus S, Koster R, Reimers J, et al. Membrane-covered stents: a new treatment strategy for saphenous vein graft lesions. *Cathet Cardiovasc Intervent* 2001;**53**:1–4.

JOSTENT® BiFLEX

Definition The JOSTENT® BiFlex is a balloon triggered super-elastic Nitinol stent intended for use in coronary and peripheral arteries. The shape memory alloy of Nitinol is not of special interest here, but rather its elastic properties. The design is based on a slotted tube design. The new, unique unit cell construction has a negative spring rate and a bistable function. The main difference compared to all other balloon expandable stents is that no plastic deformation occurs when expanding the stent. The stent snaps open in distinct steps. The crimped and the expanded cell have both stable shapes. The balloon is not used to bend the stent material. It only triggers the expansion: having overcome a certain point in balloon size, the stent expands itself to the next step by its immanent elastic forces.

Brief history • First animal trials in December 2000

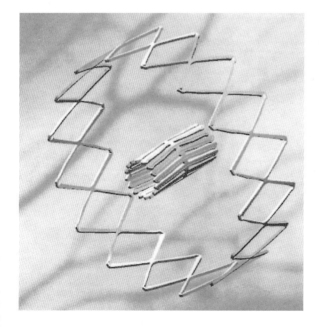

Figure 16.11: The JOSTENT® BiFlex.

139

JOSTENT® BiFlex technical specifications

Material composition:	Nitinol
Degree of radiopacity (grade):	Moderate
Feromagnetism:	None
Metallic surface area expanded:	Approx. 20% (at Ø 3 mm)
Stent design:	Slotted tube
Strut design:	Bistable cell construction
Profile(s) on the balloons:	~1 mm
Longitudinal flexibility:	Superior
Percentage shortening (on delivery):	0%
Percentage shortening on expansion:	0%
Degree of recoil (shape memory):	0%
Radial force:	High

Indications for use: as proposed by the manufacturer

Insufficient result after PTCA in the coronary vessels, e.g. residual stenosis (> 30% and/or a trans-stenotic mean pressure gradient > 5 mmHg), dissection, obstruction due to detached atherosclerotic plaque material or reocclusion.

17. THE LUNAR CORONARY STENT SYSTEM

InFlow Dynamics AG, Munich, Germany

Franz R Eberli and Stephan Windecker

Definition	Starflex design is a homogeneous, multicellular stent structure with alternating stiff and flex segments for excellent longitudinal flexibility; the Niobium alloy stent is coated with iridium oxide, which facilitates the growth of endothelial cells and reduces the inflammatory response to stent mediated vascular injury.

History	• September 2000, CE mark received • December 2000, clinical evaluation at Swiss Cardiovascular Center, Bern, Switzerland • March 2001, multicenter registry study 'Moonlight' with six European centres • March 2001, first live case with lunar coronary stent system from Inselspital, Bern, Switzerland, to Percutaneous Endovascular Therapeutics Congress, Santa Fé, Argentina

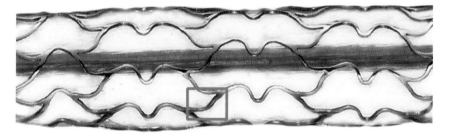

Figure 17.1: *Expanded unmounted Lunar® coronary stent. Insert shows the magnified surface.*

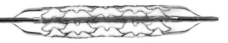

Figure 17.2: *Balloon mounted Lunar® coronary stent.*

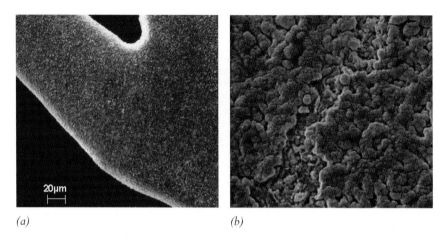

(a)   (b)

Figure 17.3: *(a) Electron microscopy of Lunar® stent. (b) Electron microscopy of Lunar stent surface showing the particularly rough surface structure of the iridium oxide coated stent. It is assumed that the iridium oxide coated, rough surface facilitates adhesion and growth of endothelial cells.*

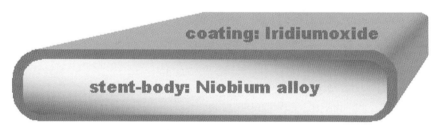

Figure 17.4: *Schematic cross-sectional drawing highlighting the special construction of the Lunar stent. The Niobium core of the stent is covered with the iridium oxide. The Niobium alloy is a heavy-metal-free material, with the same mechanical features as steel. This corrosion-free clinically proven material has self-healing features. The iridium oxide decreases the formation of free oxygen radicals, and thus decreases the inflammatory stimulus after stent implantation.*

142

Lunar stent technical specifications

Material composition:	Niobium alloy stent body iridium oxide coated
Degree of radiopacity (grade):	Superior
Ferromagnetism:	Non-ferromagnetic
MRI:	MRI-proof
Metallic surface area:	Dependent on expanded diameter (13–19%)
Stent design:	Homogeneous, multicellular stent structure, 'Starflex' – design
Strut design:	Oval strut cross-section
Strut dimensions:	90 × 85 µm
Strut angles:	Dependent on diameter
Strut thickness:	90 µm
Crossing profile(s) on the balloons:	2.5 mm balloon diameter: 0.0382 inch = 0.96 mm 4.0 balloon diameter: 0.0471 inch = 1.20 mm
Longitudinal flexibility:	Good
Percentage shortening (on delivery):	0%
Percentage shortening on expansion:	<3%
Expansion range:	2.5–4.5 mm
Degree of recoil (shape memory):	<3%
Radial force:	High
Currently available diameters:	2.5–4.0 mm
Currently available lengths Mounted/implanted Unmounted:	8 mm*, 12 mm, 16 mm, 20 mm, 24 mm*, 32 mm
Currently available sizes:	Each length for 2.5/3.0/3.5/4.0 mm balloon diameter
Recrossability of implanted stent:	Excellent
Other non-coronary types available	Peripheral stents Antares Endovascular OTW Antares Renal RX

* Planned

143

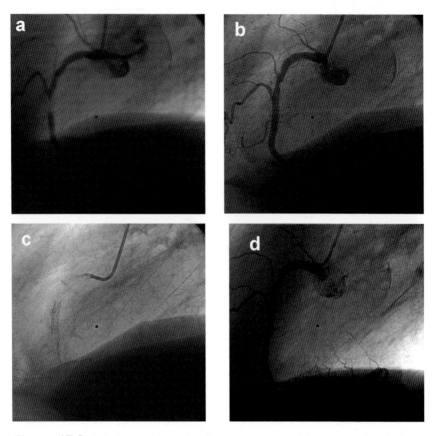

Figure 17.5: *A stenosis in the mid-right coronary artery (a) was treated with the Lunar® coronary stent (b). Fluoroscopy reveals the high radiopacity of the Lunar® stent (c). At 6 months, follow-up angiography shows an excellent late result with minimal restenosis (d).*

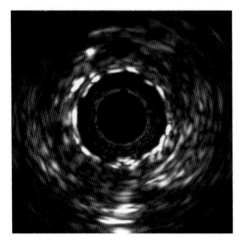

Figure 17.6: *IVUS image of a fully deployed Lunar® stent.*

Indications for use

- In patients eligible for balloon angioplasty with symptomatic ischemic heart disease characterized by discrete de novo and restenosed coronary artery lesions with reference vessel diameter from 2.5 mm to 4.5 mm.
- In elective implantation and in treatment of acute or threatened closure associated with a coronary intervention, including saphenous vein grafts.

Why I like this stent

Conceptual considerations: The Lunar® Coronary Stent System consists of a Niobium alloy stent body and a layer of homogeneous iridium oxide. The Niobium alloy is a heavy-metal-free material, with the same mechanical features as steel, but with excellent visibility. This corrosion-free clinically proven material has self-healing features.

The Lunar® coronary stent system special coating consists of a layer of ductile gold and a top layer of homogeneous iridium oxide. The gold coating assures fissure-free deployment and is also responsible for the excellent visibility of the stent. The iridium oxide coating is believed to reduce in-stent restenosis by decreasing the inflammatory response to the stent via its antioxidant action. A metallic stent induces a leucocyte reponse as soon as it is deployed. The leucoytes release hydrogen peroxide (H_2O_2), which stimulates the proliferation of vascular smooth muscle cells both directly via the activation of NF-κB, or indirectly via the formation of peroxynitrite. Iridium oxide has high catalytic properties, and cleaves H_2O_2 into water and oxygen. Therefore, the release and activation of free radicals, which provoke smooth muscle cell growth, is reduced. Experimentally, iridium oxide reduced by 50% free radical formation by stimulated leucocytes adherent to stent struts. Iridium oxide layers form a rough surface. Experimentally, adhesion of endothelial cells to the rough stent surface was markedly increased as compared to a smooth stent surface. In summary, the iridium oxide coating may promote endothelial coverage of the implanted stent while reducing free oxygen radical formation and the inflammatory response, thus reducing smooth muscle cell proliferation and in-stent restenosis. This stent property is maintained over time. The iridium oxide coating is not degraded. Therefore, the Lunar stent is not a drug eluting stent, whose effects are time-dependent.

Tips and tricks for delivery

The low profile of the Lunar stent allows easy delivery through 5 Fr guiding catheter systems. The crimping is adequate. The stent delivery system is suitable for direct stenting, but extremely tortuous vessels and calcification should be avoided.

Ongoing studies

- Moonlight study: European prospective, multicentre registry of 120 consecutive patients with single or multivessel disease. Follow-up 1 and 6 months. Started March 2001.
- Clinical evaluation of the Lunar coronary stent system at the Swiss Cardiovascular Center, Bern, Switzerland
- Clinical evaluation of the Lunar coronary stent system in Argentina and Brazil, with 40 patients.

146

18. THE MANEO STENT

DEVON Medical, Hamburg, Germany

Lutz Freiwald

Definition	The Maneo stent is a further development of PURA-VARIO-A. Its altering strut dimensions deliver excellent radiopacity and flexibility. Special crimping technology gives the stent a firm setting on the balloon and therefore makes it a safe stent implantation system.

History	After successful evaluation of this improvement in stent technology, the Maneo has been established as a 'working horse' for daily use in all proven indications.

Description	• Balloon expandable stent • Multicellular design • Segments connected with multiple links

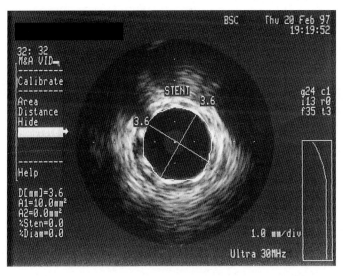

Figure 18.1: IVUS of a 16 mm long Maneo (excellent equal expansion).

Maneo coronary stent technical specifications

Material composition:	316L stainless steel
Degree of radiopacity (grade):	Excellent
Ferromagnetism:	Non-ferromagnetic
MRI:	MRI safe (details refer to IFU)

Metallic surface area
  expanded:
  unexpanded:
	Approx. 18% depending on expansion diameter.

Stent design:	Multicellular slotted tube, special round edge polishing.
Strut design:	Altering round and oval
Strut dimensions:	Altering from 0.80 to 0.150 mm
Strut thickness:	Altering from 0.80 to 0.120 mm

Profile(s):
  non expanded (uncrimped):
  expanded:
  on the balloons:
	Less than 1.1 mm

Longitudinal flexibility:	Very good
Percentage shortening on expansion:	Up to 5% depending on diameter.
Expansion range:	2.5 to 4.5 mm
Degree of recoil (shape memory):	Less than 2%
Radial force:	Excellent
Currently available diameters:	2.5, 3.0, 3.5 and 4.0 mm

Currently available lengths
  mounted/implanted:
  unmounted:
	10, 16, 24 mm
	N/A

Currently available sizes:	2.5, 3.0, 3.5 and 4.0 mm balloons with 10, 16, 24 mm stent lengths
Recrossability of implanted stent:	Excellent
Other coronary types available:	Yes. PURA-A, PURA-VARIO, PURA-VARIO-A.
Other non-coronary types available:	Yes. SAXX peripheral stent. Distributed by Bard peripheral systems.

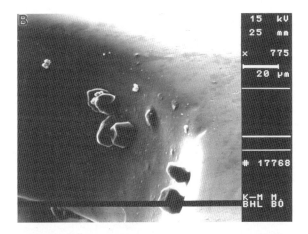

Figure 18.2: Surface polish detail of Maneo.

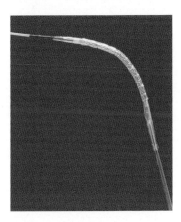

Figure 18.3: Maneo stent implantation system details (smooth balloon tip and stent-balloon conformity at the edges).

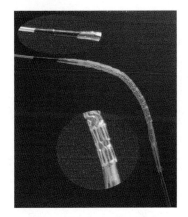

Figure 18.4: Smooth strut transition of Maneo.

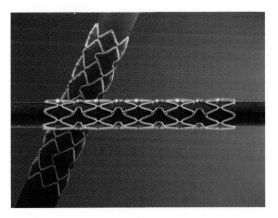

Figure 18.5: Maneo expanded to 2.5 and 3.5 mm.

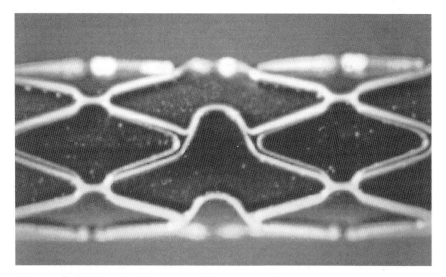

Figure 18.6: Detail of Maneo stent (altering strut dimensions).

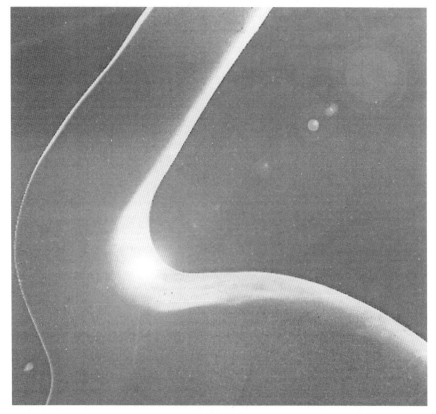

Figure 18.7: Polished surface of Maneo.

Tips and tricks for delivery

Basically the Maneo does not need tips or tricks for delivery. It is easy to use like a PTCA catheter for all currently proven indications. It is radiopaque, flexible and firmly fixed on the balloon. Therefore, the Maneo stent implantation system (SIS) can be seen as a daily 'work horse' for easy stent deployment.

Indications for use

All currently proven indications (details refer to IFU).

Why I like my stent

The Maneo is a balanced stent according to today's requirements. The stent implantation system features low compliance and high pressure. That makes the Maneo an excellent choice for daily stent procedures.

Ongoing or planned trials

Currently several trials are ongoing.

19. THE MED-X FLEXY STENT

Med-Xcor, Trévoux, France

Jean-Marie Lefebvre

Description   The Med-X Flexy stents are laser cut tubular 316 L stainless steel stents. After a first generation with closed cell design and multiple sinusoidal hinge points, a second generation was developed with improved flexibility and very low profile. More suitable for tortuous, distal or small diameter lesions, the articulation points between the cells have been reduced to one and in order to keep good radial support 2 range of cells have been added. Radiopacity is guaranteed by two golden markers at both ends of the stents allowing precise positioning and easy angiography follow-up.

History

- Beginning 1997 Development and testing
- October 1997 First clinical implantation
- End 1997–1998 Multicenter study
- November 1998 CE mark approval
  Release on the market of the bare and premounted version
- April 1999 EN46001 certification
- April 2000 Flexy stent with golden markers

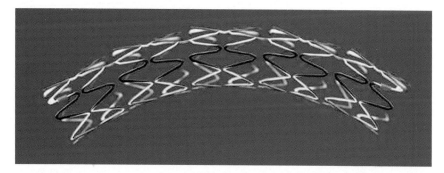

Figure 19.1: Med-X Flexy expanded stent.

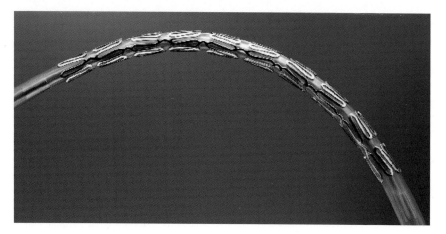

Figure 19.2: Med-X Flexy premounted stent.

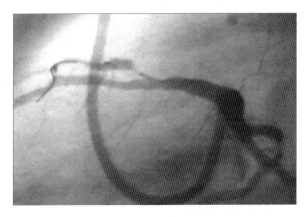

(a)

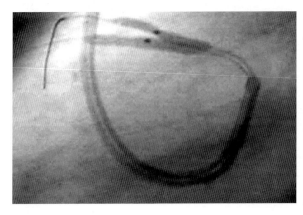

(b)

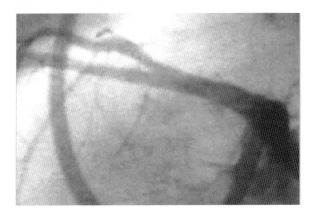

(c)

Figure 19.3: Med-X stent in bifurcated and distal lesion. (a) Final result. The Med-X stent is particularly indicated in this type of complex lesion due to its low metal coverage. (b) Angiography shows a lesion at the bifurcation including LAD and the ostium of the first diagonal. (c) A kissing balloon angioplasty technique was performed but there remains a significant stenosis. Two Med-X stents were inserted using the <Y> technique and simultaneous inflation over a 2 mm balloon for the first diagonal and a 2.5 mm balloon for the LAD. The stents were deployed at 8 atm.

Med-X stent new generation technical specifications

Material composition:	316L stainless steel
Degree of radiopacity (grade):	Excellent (markers on the stent)
Ferromagnetism:	Non-ferromagnetic (MRI safe)
Metallic surface area (metal: artery expanded):	13%
Stent design:	Zigzag rings with few articulation points
Strut design:	Rectangular with polished edge
Strut dimensions:	0.003 inch (0.07 mm) thick 0.004 inch (0.10 mm) wide
Delivery profile (crossing profile):	< 0.04 inch (< 1.0 mm)
Longitudinal flexibility:	High
Percentage shortening on expansion:	< 5%
Radial strength:	Good
Currently available diameters:	2.5, 3.0, 3.5, 4.0 mm
Currently available lengths:	8, 13, 17, 26 mm
Recrossability of implanted stent:	Excellent
Available bare (unmounted):	No
Other non-coronary types:	Peripheral stent

Med-X rapid exchange delivery system

Mechanism of deployment:	Balloon expandable
Minimal internal diameter of guiding catheter:	0.064 inch (1.6 mm), 6 Fr
Premounted on delivery catheter:	Yes
Protective sheath:	No
Position of radiopaque markers:	Proximal and distal to stent
Further balloon expansion recommended:	No
Balloon compliance:	Nominal at 8 atm
Rated burst pressure of balloon:	16 atm

Tips and tricks for delivery

There are no particular tips for delivery.

The stent is expanded fully at low pressure (around 3–4 bar), the role of increasing pressure depends upon the characteristics of the balloon.

Indications for use

*   De novo or restenotic native coronary artery and venous bypass graft stenosis
*   Suboptimal PTCA results
*   Failed PTCA

Why I like the Med-X stent

The first Med-X stent was developed with the idea of decreasing restenosis by addressing two factors: decreasing arterial wall injury and shear stress around the stent. The low quantity of metal, thin struts and favourable surface properties should reduce the activation of platelets and coagulation factors and result in less thrombus formation and thus reduce neointimal proliferation. These characteristics are even more important in vessels of smaller diameter. In addition, the manufacturing process (thermic treatment) of the Med-X stent allows for the avoidance of high pressure inflation. Lower pressure limits the stress around the vessel wall and potentially reduces neointimal proliferation. These features also result in a stent which has very good conformability ansd safe crimping capacity. This concept of a low injury stent needs, however, to be demonstrated in a large series of patients. With its second generation device, Med-Xcor wanted to maintain the benefits of the first generation device, yet improve upon the flexibility in order to meet the requirements of users who want a stent with excellent deliverability. This deliverability is a combination of three parameters: flexibility, profile and trackability. The new design of the Med-X stent with one articulation and an increased number of cells provides a compromise between excellent flexibility and good radial support. It can be used in more distal and tortuous lesions. Now the Med-X Flexy stents are available with golden markers on the stent to help precise and safe positioning in case of ostial or lesion in bifurcations.

157

Clinical trials

CE mark study: Multicenter study: $n = 60$ patients at five centers. Indications for stenting were restenosis (7.5%), dissection (32.5%) and sub-optimal PTCA results (60%).

Endpoints: Primary technical and clinical success – freedom from complications at 30 days and 6 months – 6 months angiographic and clinical status.

6 months results: Restenosis: 16%, TLR: 15%.

Open registry: 150 patients with 6 months follow-up – restenosis 13.7% – TLR: 10.4%

20. The Medtronic AVE Modular Stents – S7 and S660

Medtronic AVE, Inc., Santa Rosa, CA, USA

Eulogio Garcia

Description	Balloon-expandable, modular design with radiopaque, ellipto-rectangular struts. S7, the seventh generation of modular stent technology, is designed for 3–4 mm vessels and has a 1 mm element and 10 crown design. S660 is specifically designed for small vessels having a 1.5 mm element length and 6 crown design. Both S7 and S660 incorporate two proven Medtronic AVE delivery technologies – Discrete Technology™ for precise alignment of the stent on the balloon and Secure Technology™ to ensure stent security.

History	• October 1994 – AVE began sales of its MicroStent coronary stent line • May 2000–S660 small vessel stent released • April 2001–S7 seventh generation modular stent released

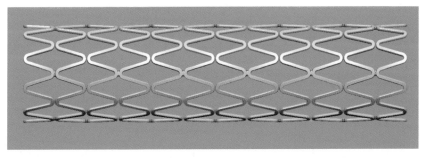

Figure 20.1: The S7 design provides an optimal balance of both deliverability and scaffolding.

Medtronic AVE S7 technical specifications

Material composition:	316 L stainless steel
Degree of radiopacity (grade):	Moderate
Ferromagnetism:	Non-ferromagnetic (MRI safe)
MRI:	MRI compatible*
Vessel wall coverage	18–24%
Stent design:	Modular, sinusoidal ring, 10 crown element design
Strut design:	Ellipto-rectangular electropolished
Strut dimensions:	1 mm long stent elements
Strut thickness:	0.004 inch × 0.005 inch
Longitudinal flexibility:	Excellent
Percentage shortening on expansion:	< 2%
Degree of recoil (shape memory):	~ 2%
Radial force:	High
Currently available diameters:	3.0–4.0 mm
Currently available lengths:	9, 12, 15, 18, 24, 30 mm
Recrossability of implanted stent:	Excellent
Other non-coronary types available:	Renal, iliac neurovascular

*Magnetic resonance imaging should not be performed until the implanted stent has been completely endothelialized (8 weeks) in order to minimize the risk of stent migration under a strong magnetic field. The stent may cause artefacts in MRI scans due to the distortion of the magnetic field.

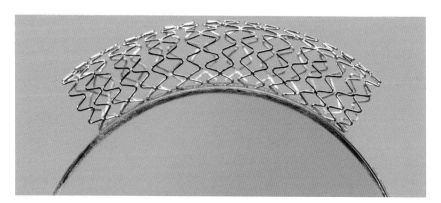

Figure 20.2: The S7 stent deployed on a bend.

Medtronic AVE S660 technical specifications

Material composition:	316 L stainless steel
Degree of radiopacity (grade):	Moderate
Ferromagnetism:	Non-ferromagnetic (MRI safe)
MRI:	MRI compatible*
Vessel wall coverage	20%
Stent design:	Modular, sinusoidal ring, 6 crown element design
Strut design:	Ellipto-rectangular electropolished
Strut dimensions:	1 mm long stent elements
Strut thickness:	0.005 inch × 0.006 inch
Profile(s): non-expanded	0.039 inch
Longitudinal flexibility:	Excellent
Percentage shortening on expansion:	~ 1.5%
Degree of recoil (shape memory):	~ 2%
Radial force:	High
Currently available diameters:	2.5 mm
Currently available lengths:	9, 12, 15, 18, 24 mm
Recrossability of implanted stent:	Excellent

*Magnetic resonance imaging should not be performed until the implanted stent has been completely endothelialized (8 weeks) in order to minimize the risk of stent migration under a strong magnetic field. The stent may cause artefacts in MRI scans due to the distortion of the magnetic field.

161

Medtronic AVE S7 rapid exchange delivery system (outside US only)

Mechanism of deployment:	Balloon expandable
Minimal internal diameter of guiding catheter:	0.064 inch
Monorail system:	Yes
Balloon characteristics:	Semi-compliant
Balloon material:	Pronto™
Guidewire lumen:	0.014 inch
Minimum recommended guide:	6 Fr
Premounted on delivery catheter:	Yes
Premounted on a high pressure balloon:	No
Protective sheath/cover:	No
Offered as a bare stent:	No
Position of radiopaque markers:	Proximal and distal to stent
Rated burst pressure of the balloon:	16 atm
Delivery balloon compliance:	Less compliant at high pressure
Longitudinal flexibility:	Excellent
Recommended deployment pressure:	Nominal at 9 atm
Further balloon expansion recommended:	Discretionary
Balloon dilatation and stent sizing:	Versatile – stent diameter dependent upon balloon diameter
Recrossability of implanted stent (grade):	Excellent
Sizing diameter:	3.0–4.0 mm

Medtronic AVE S660 rapid exchange delivery system (outside US only)

Mechanism of deployment:	Balloon expandable
Minimal internal diameter of guiding catheter:	0.064 inch
Monorail system:	Yes
Balloon characteristics:	Semi-compliant
Balloon material:	Pronto™
Guidewire lumen:	0.014 inch
Minimum recommended guide:	6 Fr
Premounted on delivery catheter:	Yes
Premounted on a high pressure balloon:	No
Protective sheath/cover:	No
Offered as a bare stent:	No
Position of radiopaque markers:	Proximal and distal to stent
Rated burst pressure of the balloon:	16 atm
Delivery balloon compliance:	Semi-compliant
Delivery profile:	0.039 inch
Longitudinal flexibility:	Excellent
Recommended deployment pressure:	Nominal at 8 atm
Further balloon expansion recommended:	Discretionary
Balloon dilatation and stent sizing:	Versatile – stent diameter dependent upon balloon diameter
Recrossability of implanted stent (grade):	Excellent
Sizing diameter:	2.5 mm

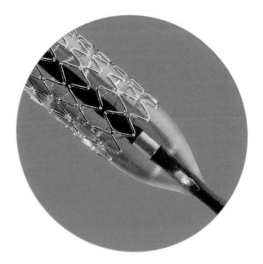

Figure 20.3: Close-up of distal stent expanded on delivery system, demonstrating the precise matching of stent length to balloon length.

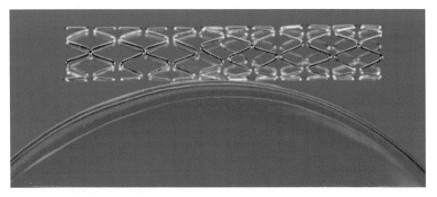

Figure 20.4: The S660 stent, uniquely designed for small vessels.

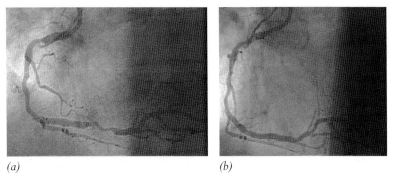

(a)   (b)

Figure 20.5: (a) S660 Pre-procedure. (b) S660 Post-procedure.

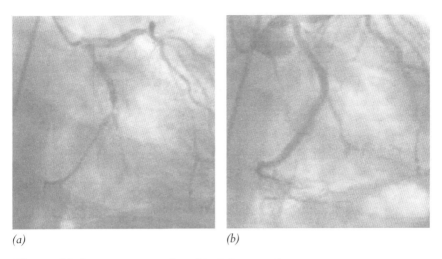

(a)   *(b)*

Figure 20.6: *(a) S7 Pre-procedure. (b) S7 Post-procedure.*

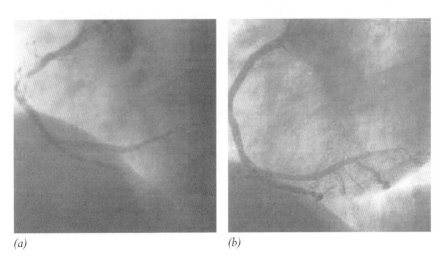

(a)   *(b)*

Figure 20.7: *(a) S7 Pre-procedure. (b) S7 Post-procedure.*

Indications for use

Elective PTCA	De novo lesions
Native coronaries and vein grafts	Restenotic lesions
Bailout	Ostial lesions
Bifurcations	Long lesions
Small vessels	Tortuous lesions

Why I like my stent
- High flexibility
- Exceptional trackability
- Optimal scaffolding
- Moderate radiopacity
- Designed for direct stenting
- Smooth, edgeless design
- Open cell design for optimal side-branch preservation and treatment
- High radial strength and low recoil to maximize MLD
- Smooth clean angiographic appearance, conforming to the vessels's natural curvature

---

Review of Current Modular Stent Literature

The interventional cardiology community now has 7 years' experience with modular stent technology, first commercialized in October 1994 by Medtronic AVE. During this period, improvements have been made in deliverability and scaffolding properties with each successive generation. These improvements have continued with the latest, seventh, the S7 Coronary Stent System.

Considerable data have been presented at global cardiology conferences indicating that the stent design has no correlation to restenosis rates. In a 1998 AHA paper, Dr Kalen Ho and Dr Richard Kuntz wrote, "Multivariate logistical regression modeling indicated that post-procedure in-stent MLD and lesion length were independent predictors of angiographic restenosis.[1] Total stent length and diabetes were of borderline statistical significance with no effect of stent type." Therefore, when choosing stents, it is necessary to refer to both the literature and the experience of other physicians who have found no statistical difference in restenosis rates among various stent designs. It may be more pertinent for a physician to select a stent that they are most

166

comfortable with regarding deliverability and scaffolding properties, e.g. a stent that can track to a lesion and treat with confidence.

The greatest testament to the effect of continuous improvement of scaffolding and deliverability in modular stents is the Restenosis and Clinical Evaluation in Coronary Arteries (RACECAR) study. The RACECAR study yielded a 6-month binary angiographic restenosis rate of 13.4 percent. Other recent literature that highlights deliverability and scaffolding optimization in modular stents and its positive effects upon acute and long-term outcomes are as follows:

1. Ho KKL, Senerchia C, Orlando R, Chuahan MS, Kuntz RE. Medical Center, Boston, MA, Predictors of angiographic restenosis after stenting: pooled analysis of 1,197 patients with protocol-mandated angiographic follow-up from 5 randomized stent trials, Abstract, 71st AHA scientific session, 1998.

2. Schalij MJ, Lucas H, Savalle LH, Tresukosol D, Jukema JW, Reiber JHC, Bruschke AVG. Micro Stent I, initial results, and six months follow-up by quantative coronary angiography. *Cathet Cardiovasc Diagn* 1998;**43**:19–27

3. Oemrawsingh PV, Tuinenburg JC, Schalij MJ, Jukema JW, Reiber HC, Bruschke VG. Clinical and angiographic outcome of Microstent II implantation in native coronary arteries. *Am J Cardiol* 1998;**81**:152–7.

4. Haase J, Geimer M, Gohrings S, Kerkar P, Agrawal R, Storger H, Preusier W, Schawartz F, Reifart N. Results of Micro Stent implantations in coronary lesions of various complexity. *Am J Cardiol* 1997;**80**:1601–2.

5. Agarwal R, Bhargava B, Kaul U et al. Long-term outcome of intracoronary microstent implantation: lesion-matched comparison with Palmaz-Schatz stent [see comments]. *Cathet Cardiovasc Diagn* 1998;**43**:397–401.

6. Eeckhout E, Groberty M, Vogt P et al. Corrective use of the 2.5-mm GFX stent for suboptimal angioplasty results in small coronary arteries. *Cathet Cardiovasc Intervent* 1999;**48**:157–61.

7. Koster R, Terres W, Hamm C, Kahler J, Meinertz T. Initial clinical and angiographic results with the AVE Micro-Stent. *Z Kardiol* 1996;**85**:640–6.

21. THE MEGAflex CORONARY STENT

EuroCor GmbH, Bonn, Germany

Israel Tamari and Michael Orlowski

Description	• Balloon expandable tubular stent • Multicellular, modular ring design • Alternating connections with multiple links • Optimized, spring alike expansion force for maximized intrastent luminal gain • Unique, unsurpassed flexibility for angulated stenting in > 180° vessel morphologies • Conformability 1:1 stent to artery morphology. The MEGAflex is designed for tortuous vessels, in particular for stenting lesions in the ramus circumflexus • Special surface polishing technique guarantees low thrombogenicity

History	• December 2000 – first MEGAflex human implants in Germany, Israel, Austria and India • European CE mark approval received • End of February 2001–1400 MEGAflex human implants

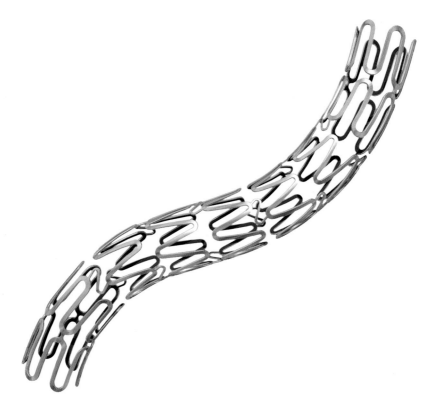

Figure 21.1: *Genius MEGAflex® coronary stent.*

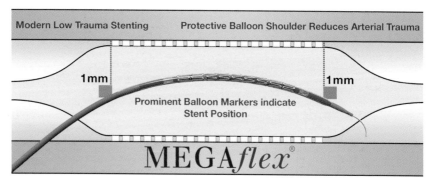

Figure 21.2: *MEGAflex® low trauma stenting.*

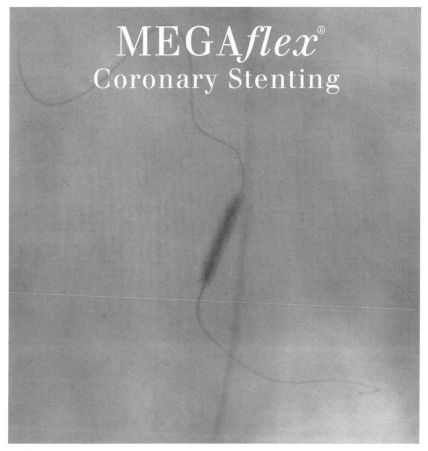

Figure 21.3: MEGAflex coronary stent.

MEGAflex stent technical specifications

Material composition:	316 L stainless steel
Degree of radiopacity:	Excellent
Ferromagnetism:	Non-ferromagnetic (MRI safe)
Metal surface area (metal: artery, expanded):	18–20%
Stent design:	Multicellular-modular ring design Alternating connections with multiple links
Strut design:	Tubular, smooth rounded
Strut dimensions:	0.004 inch (0.11 mm) thick
Profile: non-expanded (uncrimped):	1.6 mm (0.06 inch)
Expanded:	up to 4.5 mm
On the balloon:	0.036 inch
Longitudinal flexibility:	High
Percentage shortening on delivery:	None
Percentage shortening on expansion:	< 3%
Expansion range:	2.5–4.0 mm
Degree of recoil (shape memory):	< 2%
Radial force (to collapse):	High, excellent
Currently available diameters:	2.5, 2.75, 3.0, 3.5 and 4.0 mm
Currently available lengths:	
Mounted	9, 11, 13, 15, 17, 19, 23, 25, 27 mm
Unmounted	9, 11, 15, 19, 23, 27 mm
Currently available sizes:	2.5–4 mm
Re-crossibility of implanted stent:	Excellent
Other non-coronary types:	None

MEGAflex coronary stent delivery system

Mechanism of deployment:	Balloon expandable
Mechanism of expanding:	Balloon expandable
Minimum internal diameter of guiding catheter:	0.064 inch (1.6 mm) 5 Fr
Monorail system:	Yes
Balloon characteristics	Semi-compliant, moderately
Balloon material:	Polyamide
Guidewire lumen:	0.014 inch (0.36 mm)
Minimum recommended guide:	5 Fr
Premounted on delivery cath:	Yes
Premounted on high pressure B:	Yes
Protected sheath cover:	Yes
Offered as a bare stent:	Yes
Position of radiopaque markers:	Proximal and distal stent ends
Rated burst pressure of balloon:	16 atm for 2.5–3.5 mm
	14 atm for 4.0 mm
Delivery balloon compliance:	Semi-compliant, moderately
Delivery profile (crossing profile):	0.036–0.038 inch
Longitudinal flexibility:	Extremely flexible
Recommended deployment pressure:	Nominal at 8 atm
Further balloon expansion recommended:	At physician's discretion
Balloon dilatation and stent sizing:	Equal to artery or up to 10%
Recrossibility of implanted stent:	Excellent
Sizing diameter:	2.5–4.5 mm

Current indications for clinical use

- Native coronary arteries, de novo and restenotic lesions
- Restensosis
- Bifurcation
- Lesions in a bend
- Ramus Circumflexus
- Suboptimal PTCA result

173

Why I like my stent

- The MEGAflex is ideal for angulated lesions. It provides a 1:1 conformity to complex vessel morphologies
- It is very good for bifurcation stenting because of the particular stent window design
- The MEGAflex expands homogenously at a very low pressure of 3 bars only
- It assures a low trauma stenting quality
- Overexpansion in order to make up for recoil is never necessary
- Full effective stent expansion at low pressures of 10 atm
- The MEGAflex is mounted on a semi-compliant balloon delivery device.
- Short balloon shoulders of 0.5–1.0 mm only reduce arterial trauma at stent expansion
- The delivery catheter provides an excellent tracking like gliding quality, without any friction due to a high density polyethylene inner lumen surface technology
- The lesion crossing profile is just 0.036 inch and ensures superb lesion crossing
- The stent can be easily advanced through stents due to its smooth and rounded strut features
- The high radial force makes the MEGAflex ideal for B2 and C lesions
- The MEGAflex is the stent for tortuous vessel anatomy

Ongoing or planned trials

CTS
Multicenter study 'Complex tortuous vessel stenting'
Number of patients   200
MEGAflex
Drug delivery stent trials
Number of patients   500

22. THE MULTI-LINK PENTA™ CORONARY STENT SYSTEM

Guidant Vascular Intervention Group, Santa Clara, CA, USA

Wim J van der Giessen and Susan Veldhof

Description	• Balloon expandable stent • Tubular design • Multiple rings connected with multiple links

History of workhorse coronary stents	*ACS Multi-Link®* • 1993 first clinical experience reported by Ulrich Sigwart • 1994 first multicentre registry study started • 1995 clinical use in Europe, Canada and Asia/Pacific • 1996 approved in Japan • 1997 approved by FDA for use in the United States *ACS Multi-Link DUET™* • 1997 CE marked. Clinical use in Europe, Canada and Asia/Pacific • 1998 approved by FDA for use in the United States *ACS Multi-Link TRISTAR™* • 1999 CE marked. Clinical use in Europe, Canada and Asia/Pacific • 1999 approved by FDA for use in the United States *ACS Multi-Link TETRA™* • 2000 CE marked. Clinical use in Europe, Canada and Asia/Pacific • 2000 approved by FDA for use in the United States *ACS Multi-Link PENTA™* • 2001 CE marked. Clinical use in Europe and Asia/Pacific • 2001 approved by FDA for use in the United States

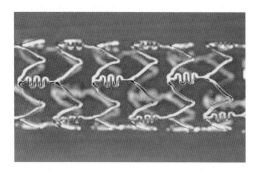

Figure 22.1 (Expanded stent): *The Multi-Link PENTA™ stent is a balloon expandable stent with the classic MULTI-LINK™ corrugated ring design. It has multiple rings connected with three links each to provide uniform scaffolding.*

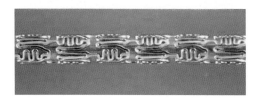

Figure 22.2 (Unexpanded stent): *New ACCESS-Link™ technology provides a significant increase in flexibility to access complex lesions. The 5-turn ACCESS-Link™ is embedded within the corrugated ring to achieve flexibility without sacrificing scaffolding.*

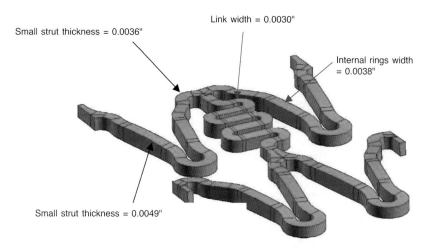

Link width = 0.0030"

Small strut thickness = 0.0036"

Internal rings width = 0.0038"

Small strut thickness = 0.0049"

Figure 22.3: *The Multi-Link PENTA™ has VTS™ technology. Struts are thin in areas where the stent needs to flex and thicker in remaining areas to maintain radiopacity and radial strength.*

176

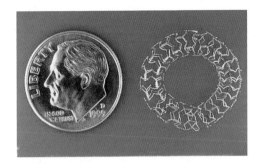

Figure 22.4: *Excellent conformability is achieved with the combination of the ACCESS-Link™ and VTS™ technologies.*

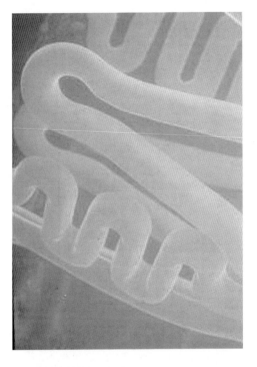

Figure 22.5: *Stent struts are electropolished to a rounded, smooth surface finish (SEM image, magnification 100×).*

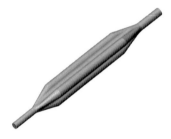

Figure 22.6: *The WRAP™ balloon technology: unique balloon shape allows for improved rewrap and lower profile upon deflation after stent expansion.*

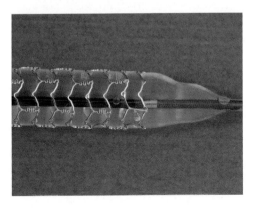

Figure 22.7: *The WRAP™ balloon with S.T.E.P™ technology: minimizes the amount of vessel dilated outside the stent. The stepped tapers provide a gradual transition from the deploying stent to the unstented vessel. Photograph of 3.0 × 18 mm expanded system at nominal pressure.*

177

Multi-Link PENTA™ stent technical specifications

Material composition:	316L stainless steel
Degree of radiopacity (grade):	Moderate
Ferromagnetism:	Non-ferromagnetic (MRI safe)
Metallic surface area (expanded):	16.9% metal-to-artery ratio at 3.0 mm diameter
Stent design:	Laser cut from a stainless steel tube. Pattern based on the traditional Guidant Multi-Link corrugated ring footprint. Each ring is connected by 3 links (3–3–3 design) that have 5 turns embedded within the ring
Strut design:	Rounded struts with VTS™ technology: an innovative technology allowing the struts to be thin where flexibility is needed and thick in other areas to provide radiopacity (VTS = variable thickness strut)
Strut dimensions:	Strut thickness (t): Small t: 0.0036 inch (0.09 mm) Large t: 0.0049 inch (0.12 mm) Strut width: Body cell: 0.0038 inch (0.10 mm) End ring: 0.0046 inch (0.12 mm)
Longitudinal flexibility:	High
Percentage shortening on expansion:	1.8% for 3.0 × 18 mm. Stent designed to be within 5% of label length at any expansion diameter
Degree of recoil (shape memory):	2.9% for 3.0 × 18 mm
Radial force:	High
Currently available diameters:	2.75, 3.0, 3.5, 4.0 mm
Expansion range:	Maximum expansion 2.75–3.0 mm diameters: 3.5 mm Maximum expansion 3.5–4.0 mm diameters: 4.5 mm
Currently available lengths:	8, 13, 15, 18, 23, 28, 33 mm
Recrossability of implanted stent:	Excellent
Other non-coronary types available:	Iliac and renal; carotid and neuro in clinical trials

Multi-Link RX PENTA™ stent delivery system

Mechanism of deployment:	Balloon expandable
Pre-mounted on delivery catheter:	Yes
Pre-mounted on a high pressure balloon:	Yes
Protective sheath/cover:	No
Monorail system:	Yes
Minimal internal diameter of guiding catheter:	0.056 inch (5F) compatible for all sizes and lengths
Balloon characteristics:	The Multi-Link PENTA™ balloon is specifically designed for deployment and deflation. It incorporates: • The WRAP™ balloon: a unique balloon shape that eases the ability of the balloon to rewrap into lower profiles upon deflation, and • S.T.E.P.™ technology: stepped balloon tapers that reduce the degree of vessel dilation outside the stent. It has been designed to minimize the potential for edge dissection. (S.T.E.P. = short transitional edge protection)
Mechanism of expanding:	The WRAP™ balloon with S.T.E.P.™ technology is tri-folded to enable even inflation and to ensure uniform stent deployment both radially and longitudinally
Balloon material:	XCELON™ (nylon)
Longitudinal flexibility:	Excellent
Position of radiopaque markers:	Proximal and distal dual, swaged markers clearly indicate both the position of the expanded stent and the balloon working length
Stent security	The stent GRIP™ process promotes excellent stent retention. It provides smooth surface transition between stent and balloon, protecting stent edges

continued

179

Multi-Link RX PENTA™ stent delivery system – continued

Delivery balloon compliance:	Nominal:	8 atm
	+¼ size:	14 atm
	RBP:	16 atm
Recommended deployment pressure:	Between 8 and 16 atm according to lesion characteristics	
Further dilatation recommended:	At physician's discretion. The stent delivery system can be used for post-dilatation	
Sizing diameter:	Matching target vessel diameter	
Delivery profile: (crossing profile)	2.75 mm	0.041 inch (1.04 mm)
	3.0 mm	0.042 inch (1.07 mm)
	3.5 mm	0.044 inch (1.12 mm)
	4.0 mm	0.046 inch (1.17 mm)

Current indications for clinical use

- Native coronary arteries, de novo and restenotic lesions

New product developments

- Multi-Link Pixel stent system – see Chapter 23
- Multi-Link Penta Grande stent system
- Bifurcation stent

On-going or planned trials

Name	Number of patients	Type	Status follow-up	Results
WEST 1	102	Registry; Full Anticoagulation	Complete; 1 year data available	Target lesion restenosis: 12% Target vessel restenosis: 17% 30 day MACE: 5.9% 6 month MACE: 17.6% 1 year MACE: 18.8%
WEST 2	165	Registry; On-line IVUS and QCA; ASA only	Complete; 6 month data available	SAT rate: 1.2% Restenosis: 12.8% 30 day MACE: 1.8% 6 month MACE: 9.1%
ASCENT	1040	Randomized Multi-Link vs Palmaz–Schatz ASA and Ticlid; de novo lesions	9 month clinical and angiographic data complete	SAT rate: 0.6% for ML vs 1.7% for PS 9 month in-stent restenosis rate: 16% for ML vs 22.1% for PS; 9 month MACE rate: 8.1% for ML vs 19.3% for PS
ASCENT Long Term Follow-Up	545	Post-approval data	3 year follow-up complete	
ASCENT Restenosis Registry	201	Registry; Primary restenosis lesions	9 month clinical follow-up complete	9 month target vessel failure rate: 15.9%; 9 month MACE: 10.4%
High ASCENT	101	Registry using RX Multi-Link HP System	30 day clinical follow-up complete	2.0% 30 day MACE rate; 78% of patients successfully post-dilated with stent system, patients discharged from hospital significantly sooner than ASCENT patients, 1.3 vs 1.6 days
Long ASCENT	202	Registry using RX Multi-Link System in 15 mm, 25 mm and 35 mm lengths	30–day clinical follow-up complete	30 day MACE rate: 3.5%

continued

181

On-going or planned trials – continued

Name	Number of patients	Type	Status follow-up	Results
IVUS	49	Registry using ML with IVUS	12 month clinical follow-up complete	12 month MACE rate: 2% significant increase in average vessel area comparing 12 atm deployment pressure to 8 atm
Japan	1123	Registry	6–month clinical and angiographic follow-up complete	In-stent restenosis 14%
CADILLAC	2000	Randomized using Multi-Link and Multi-Link Duet stenting vs PTCA in MI with ReoPro	12 month follow-up complete	MACE at 6 months; PTCA no abciximab 19.3% PTCA + abciximab 15.2% Stent no abciximab 10.8% Stent + abciximab 10.9% Other results pending
SLIDE Europe	360	Randomized using ML-Duet direct stenting (no pre-dilatation vs standard pre-dilatation strategy)	6 month clinical follow-up complete	Procedural success for direct stenting 93.8% MACE at 6 months 7.1% for direct stenting vs 6.7%
SLIDE US	250	Registry direct stenting	30 day follow-up complete; 6 month ongoing	30 day MACE 1.2% SAT 0% TVF 1.6%
AMIGO	750	Randomized using ML and ML Duet, debulk with DA + stent vs stent alone	6 month follow-up complete	In progress
DESIRE	500	Randomized using ML, debulk with DA + stent vs stent alone	In progress (Japan)	

continued

On-going or planned trials – continued

Name	Number of patients	Type	Status follow-up	Results
DUET US	270	Registry using ML Duet, de novo lesions	6 month clinical and angiographic follow-up complete	30 day MACE rate: 2.2%; 6 month TVF rate 11.9%; ML Duet significantly better vs ML (historically) in both device success (99.6% vs 97.1%) and procedure success (97.8% vs 93.9%)
DUET Europe	210	Registry; Duet stent; de novo lesions; 8–23 mm in length	6 month follow-up complete	30 day MACE rate: 4.3% 6 month MACE rate: 16.7% Restenosis rate: 16.3%
REVIVE	160	Registry using ML Duet; saphenous vein bypass lesions	6 month follow-up complete	6 month MACE 19.4% TVF 20.0% SAT 0%
SOS	1000	Randomized stenting vs CABG in multivessel disease	6 month follow-up complete	In progress
Culottes (Europe)	100	Registry; stents in bifurcation lesions	6 month follow-up complete	In progress
TETRA Registry	202	Registry, native de novo lesions 3.0–4.0 mm	6 month follow-up complete	Primary endpoint 14 day MACE 2% 6 month results pending
PENTA Registry	200	Native de novo lesions, 3.0–4.0 mm 8,13,18,23, and 28mm stents 6 month angiographic follow-up	30 day follow-up complete 6 month in progress	In hospital MACE 1.1% (first 95 patients for FDA filing)
TRENDS	1000	De novo and restenotic; randomized to pre-dilatation and no pre-dilatation. 6-month angiographic follow-up.	Enrolment in progress	

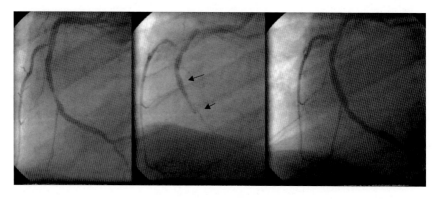

Figure 22.8: *(a) A 65-year-old male patient was admitted for PTCA of the right coronary artery 2 weeks after a non-Q-wave inferior infarction. Angiogram of the RCA showed a severe stenosis with thrombus distal. (b) It proved quite easy to attempt direct stenting of this lesion with a 3.5 × 15 mm Multi-Link Penta™ stent system (arrows). (c) A single inflation up to 12 atm proved sufficient to obtain a nice angiographic result.*

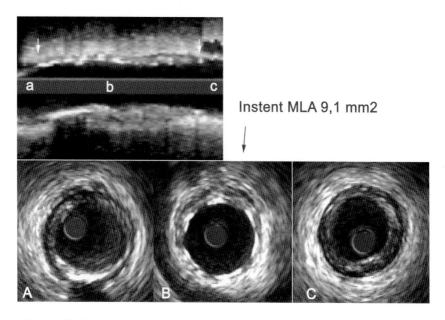

Instent MLA 9,1 mm2

Figure 22.9: *IVUS assessment of the result of direct stenting in the RCA (same patient as Figure 8). The cross-sectional images have been obtained from the sites with corresponding lettering at the longitudinal pull back. The stent shows nice apposition and symmetry. Protrusion of soft plaque material through the stent could not be observed.*

References

1. Rogers C, Edelman E. Endovascular stent design dictates experimental restenosis and thrombosis. *Circulation* 1995; **91**:2995–3001.

2. Priestley KA, Clague JA, Buller NP, Sigwart U. First clinical experience with a new, flexible, low profile metallic stent and delivery system. *Eur Heart J* 1996; **17**:438–44.

3. Emanuelsson H, Serruys PW, van der Giessen WJ, Dawkins K, Rutsch W, Katus H, Morel MA, Veldhof S, Wijns W, Sigwart U. Clinical and angiographic results with the MULTI-LINK™ – The West European Stent Trail (WEST). *J Invasive Card* 1997; **9**:561–8.

4. Serruys PW, van der Giessen W, Garcia E, Macaya, C, Colombo A, Mudra H, Fleck E, Ormiston J, Figulla H, Seabra Gomes R, Veldhof S, Morel MA for the WEST 2 Investigators. Clinical and angiographic results with the MULTI-LINK™ stent implanted under intravascular ultra sound guidance (WEST 2). *J Invasive Card* 1998; **10**:20B-27B.

5. Carrozza JP, Hermiller JB, Linnemeir TJ, Popma JJ, Yock PG, Roubin GS, Dean LS, Kuntz RE, Robertson L, Ho KK, Cutlip DE, Baim DS. Quantitative coronary angiographic and intravascular ultrasound assessment of a new nonarticulated stent: report from the advanced cardiovascular systems MULTI-LINK™ stent pilot study. *J Am Coll Cardiol* 1998; **31**:50–6.

6. Pentousis D, Guerin Y, Funck F, Zheng H, Toussaint M, Corcos T, Favereau X. Direct stent implantation without predilatation using the MULTI-LINK™ stent. *Am J Cardiol* 1998; **82**: 1437–40.

7. Keriakes D, Midei M, Hermiller J, O'Shaughnessy C, Schlofmitz R, Yakubov S, Fink S, Hu F, Nishimura N, Sievers M, Valentine ME, Broderick T, Lansky A, Moses J. Procedural and late outcome following MULTI-LINK RX DUET coronary stent deployment. *Am J Cardiol* 1999; **84**:1385–90.

8. Te Riele JAM, Piek JJ, Mudra H,Schofer J, Betrand M, Rutsch W, Beekman JA, Veldhof S, Eijgelshoven MHJ, Serruys PW. Clinical and angiographic results with the ACS Multi-Link DUET coronary stent system. The DUET Study. *Int J Cardiovasc Interven* 2000; **3**:97–104.

9. Kastrati A, Dirschinger J, Boekstegers P, Elezi S, Schuhlen H, Pache J, Steinbeck G, Schmitt C, Ulm K, Neumann FJ, Schoemig A. Influence of stent design on 1–year outcome after coronary stent placement: a randomized comparison of five stent types in 1,147 unselected patients. *Catheter Cardiovasc Interv* 2000; **50**:290–7.

10. Kereiakes D, Linnemeier TJ, Baim DS, Kuntz R, O'Shaughnessy C, Hermiller J, Fink S, Lansky A, Nishimura N, Broderick TM, Popma J. Usefulness of stent length in predicting in-stent restenosis (the MULTI-LINK stent trials). *Am J Cardiol* 2000; **86**:336–41.

11. Carter AJ, Lee DP, Suzuki T, Bailey L, Lansky A, Jones R, Virmani R. Experimental evaluation of a short transitional edge protection balloon for intracoronary stent deployment. *Cathet Cardiovasc Interven* 2000; **51**:112–19.

12. DS Baim, DE Cutlip, M Midei, TJ Linnemeier, T Schreiber, D Cox, D Kereiakes, JJ Popma, L Robertson, R Prince, AJ Lansky, KK Ho, RE Kuntz. Final results of a randomized trial comparing the MULTI-LINK stent with the Palmaz-Schatz stent for narrowings in native coronary arteries. *Am J Cardiol* 2001; **87**:157–62.

13. Foley DP, Kereiakes D, te Riele JAM, Nishimura N, Veldhof S, Fink S, Yeung A, van Hoogenhuyze D, Lansky A, van Es G-A, Kutryk MJB, Serruys PW, on behalf of the US and European DUET Investigators. Acute and 6 month clinical and angiographic outcome after implantation of the ACS Duet stent for single vessel coronary artery disease: final results of the European and US ACS Multi-Link Duet™ Registry. *Cathet Cardiovasc Interv* 2001 (in press).

23. THE MULTI-LINK RX PIXEL™ CORONARY STENT SYSTEM

Guidant, Santa Clara, CA, USA

Wim J van der Giessen and Susan Veldhof

Description	• Balloon expandable stent • Tubular design • Multiple rings connected with multiple links

History	• 2000 CE marked • Clinical use in Europe, Canada, Asia/Pacific, United States

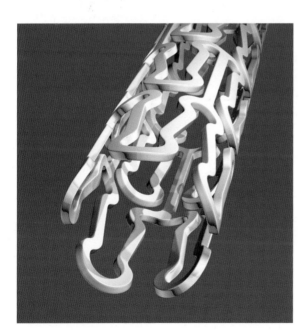

Figure 23.1: The Multi-Link PIXEL™ is a balloon expandable stent designed specifically for treating small vessels. It is a tubular 3-3-3 corrugated ring design with five crests and low strut thickness to provide high flexibility, conformability and radial strength without compromising scaffolding.

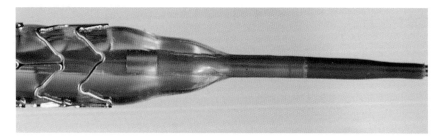

Figure 23.2: S.T.E.P.™ Balloon Technology reduces the amount of excess balloon material outside the stent and minimizes the chance for small vessel edge dissections.

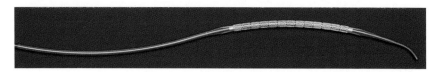

Figure 23.3: Multi-Link PIXEL™ offers low system profiles, GRIP™ Technology for stent security, proximal and distal balloon markers that indicate the position of the expanded stent and balloon working length and a lubricious Hydrocoat hydrophilic coating for improved deliverability.

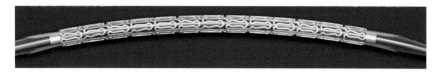

Figure 23.4: Detail of Fig. 23.3. ML Pixel crimped on delivery balloon system.

Multi-Link RX PIXEL™ stent technical specifications

Material composition:	316 L stainless steel
Degree of radiopacity (grade):	Moderate
Ferromagnetism:	Non-ferromagnetic (MRI safe)
Metallic surface area (expanded):	14% metal-to-artery ratio at 2.5 mm
Stent design:	Laser cut from a solid stainless steel tube in the corrugated ring pattern. Each ring is connected by 3-3-3 links
Strut design:	Unsupported surface area 2.0 mm² and 4.0 mm² at 2.5 mm
Strut dimensions:	Thickness: 0.0039 inch (0.099 mm) Width: 0.0038 inch (0.096 mm)
Longitudinal flexibility:	High
Percentage shortening on expansion:	1.50% (2.5 × 18 mm)
Degree of recoil (shape memory):	1.4% (2.5 × 18 mm)
Radial force:	Excellent. Full collapse at 46 psi (2.5 size)
Currently available diameters:	2.0, 2.25, 2.5 mm
Expansion range:	Maximum expansion 3.0 mm
Currently available lengths: RX PIXEL:	8, 13, 18, 23, 28 mm

Multi-Link RX PIXEL™ stent delivery system

Mechanism of deployment:	Balloon expandable
Pre-mounted on delivery catheter:	Yes
Pre-mounted on a high pressure balloon:	Yes
Protective sheath/cover:	No
Monorail system:	Yes
Minimal internal diameter of guiding catheter:	0.056 inch (5 Fr) compatible for all sizes and lengths
Balloon characteristics:	The Multi-Link PIXEL balloon is specifically designed for stent delivery. It incorporates S.T.E.P.™* technology, a unique design that reduces the amount of balloon material outside the stent. It is designed to minimize the potential for edge dissection. *Short Transitional Edge Protection
Mechanism of expanding:	The S.T.E.P.™ balloon design with tri-fold enables even inflation pressure and ensures uniform stent deployment both radially and longitudinally.
Balloon material:	XCELON™ (nylon)
Position of radiopaque markers:	Proximal and distal markers clearly indicate both the position of the expanded stent and the balloon working length.
Recommended deployment pressure:	Between 7 and 16 atm according to lesion characteristics.
Delivery balloon compliance:	2.25 and 2.5 mm sizes nominal: 7 atm +1/4 size: 16 atm R.B.P.: 16 atm 2.0 mm size nominal: 7 atm + 1/4 size: 20 atm R.B.P.: 20 atm
Further dilatation recommended:	At physician's discretion. The stent delivery system can be used for post-dilatation.

Sizing diameter:	Matching target vessel diameter
Delivery profile (crossing profile):	2.0 mm 0.036 inch (0.91 mm)
	2.25 mm 0.036 inch (0.91 mm)
	2.5 mm 0.037 inch (0.94 mm)

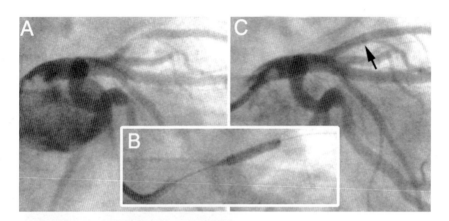

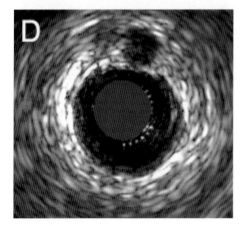

Figure 23.5: *(a) Male patient, 47 years of age, presented with unstable angina and a subtotal lesion in a 2.5 mm first diagonal branch. (b) Using direct stenting technique the lesion was crossed with 2.5 × 13 mm ML Pixel stent system, which was inflated for 50 seconds up to 12 atm. (c) Good acute angiographic result. (d) IVUS examination showed good apposition and symmetric expansion of the Pixel stent (this echo frame was recorded at the site of the arrow in Fig. 23.5c).*

On-going or planned trials

Name	Number of patients	Type	Status/follow-up	Results
PIXEL™ (US)	150	Registry using ML PIXEL, for abrupt threatened closure in de novo or restenotic lesions in vessels 2.0 mm to 2.5 mm	30 day primary endpoint completed; 6 months secondary endpoint in progress	30 day MACE 0.7% TVF rate 1.3% SAT 0.7% 6 months pending
PIXEL™ (Europe and India)	360	Randomized trial pre dilatation vs direct stenting with 6 month angiographic follow up in de novo and restenotic lesions in vessels sized ≥ 2.2 mm − ≤ 2.7 mm	Study initiation in progress	

Current indications for clinical use
* Designed specifically for small vessel lesions

192

24. THE MULTI-LINK RX ULTRA™ CORONARY STENT SYSTEM

Guidant – Advanced Cardiovascular Systems, Inc, Santa Clara, CA, USA

Wim J van der Giessen and Susan Veldhof

Description	• Balloon expandable stent • Tubular design • Multiple rings connected with multiple links

History	• 1999 CE marked. • Clinical use in Europe, Canada, Asia/Pacific • 2000 FDA approval for use in United States

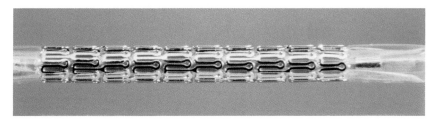

Figure 24.1(a): *The balloon-expandable Multi-Link RX Ultra™ is available premounted. A new crimping technique offers better retention to the balloon.*

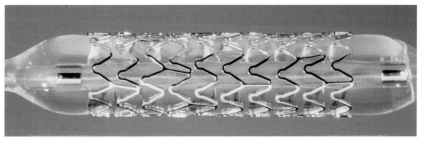

Figure 24.1(b): *The Multi-Link RX Ultra™ may be especially useful for stenting of friable lesions due to its higher metal-to-artery ratio.*

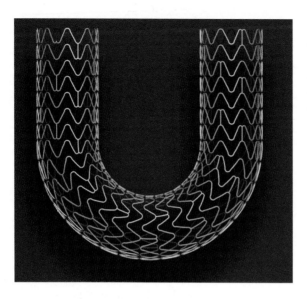

Figure 24.1(c): *The Multi-Link Ultra™ combines flexibility with radial force, two factors important for use in saphenous vein grafts.*

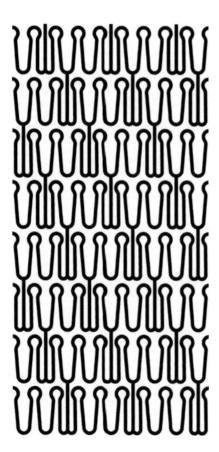

Figure 24.1(d): *The basic structure of the Multi-Link Ultra™ is similar to other members of the Multi-Link family, but the Ultra™ contains more interconnecting links per surface area.*

194

Multi-Link RX Ultra™ stent technical specifications

Material composition:	316L stainless steel
Degree of radiopacity (grade):	Moderate
Ferromagnetism:	Non-ferromagnetic (MRI safe)
Metallic surface area (expanded):	19% metal-to-artery ratio at 3.5 mm
Stent design:	Laser cut from a solid stainless steel tube in the corrugated ring pattern. Each ring is connected by 3–3–3 links
Strut design:	Proprietary. Unsupported surface area 3.8 mm^2 at 3.5 mm
Strut dimensions: thickness:	0.0050 inch (0.13 mm)
width:	0.0040 inch (0.10 mm)
Longitudinal flexibility:	Moderate/high
Percentage shortening on expansion:	2.70% (4.5 × 28 mm)
Degree of recoil (shape memory):	1.70% (4.5 × 28 mm)
Radial force:	Excellent. Full collapse at 50 psi
Currently available diameters:	3.5, 4.0, 4.5, 5.0 mm
Expansion range:	Maximum expansion 5.5 mm
Currently available lengths:	13, 18, 28, 38 mm

Multi-Link RX Ultra™ stent delivery system

Mechanism of deployment:	Balloon expandable
Pre-mounted on delivery catheter:	Yes
Pre-mounted on a high pressure balloon:	Yes
Protective sheath/cover:	No
Monorail system:	Yes
Minimal internal diameter of guiding catheter:	3.5–4.5 mm: 0.066 inch (6Fr) compatible for all lengths 5.0 mm: 0.075 inch (7Fr) compatible for all lengths
Balloon characteristics:	The Multi-Link Ultra balloon is specifically designed for stent delivery. It is not available as a dilatation balloon
Mechanism of expanding:	Tri-fold balloon to distribute even inflation pressure and ensure concentric stent deployment
Balloon material:	XCELON™ (nylon)
Position of radiopaque markers:	Proximal and distal markers indicate balloon working length
Recommended deployment pressure:	Between 9 and 14 atm according to lesion characteristics
Minimum deployment pressure:	9 atm
Rated burst pressure of balloon:	14 atm
Further dilatation recommended:	At physician's discretion. The stent delivery system can be used for post-dilatation
Sizing diameter:	Matching target vessel diameter
Delivery profile:	3.5 mm 0.056 inch (0.14 mm) 4.0 mm 0.057 inch (0.14 mm) 4.5 mm 0.057 inch (0.14 mm) 5.0 mm 0.057 inch (0.14 mm)

On-going or planned trials

Name	Number of patients	Type	Status follow-up	Results
ULTRA REVIVE SVG	194	Registry using ML ULTRA, saphenous vein bypass graft lesions	30 day and 6 month follow-up complete	30 day MACE 12.0% TVF 12.0% SAT 0.5% 6 months pending
ULTRA REVIVE De Novo	100	Registry using ML ULTRA, de novo, native coronary artery lesions	30 day and 6 month follow-up complete	30 day MACE 4.0% Post-procedure % diameter stenosis 6.9% 6 months pending

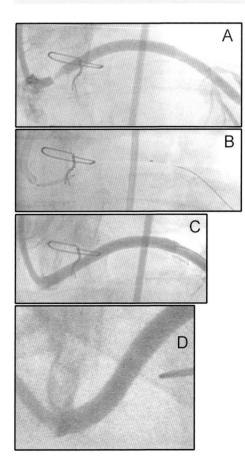

Figure 24.2: Multi-Link RX Ultra patient: A. Short proximal graft disease (13-year-old SVG) with hazy angiographic appearance. B. Direct stenting with Multi-Link RX Ultra (4.5 mm diameter, 13 mm length). C. Good acute angiographic result.
D. Magnified angio-frame shows smooth edges without signs of tissue protrusion.

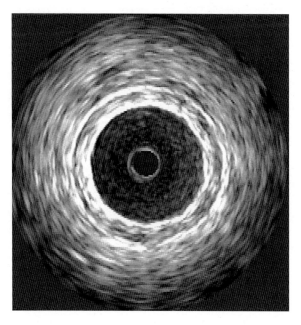

Figure 24.3: *Bail out stenting for a flow-limiting dissection after balloon angioplasty in a large right coronary artery. A 5.0 × 18 mm Multi-Link RX Ultra was placed successfully with a maximal inflation pressure of 14 atm. IVUS showed complete covering of the dissection by the stent. Complete, symmetrical deployment is one of the nice features of this stent.*

Current indications for clinical use

- Designed specifically for saphenous vein graft lesions

25. THE NEXUS AND NEXUS II CORONARY STENTS

Occam International BV, Eindhoven, The Netherlands

Thomas A Ischinger and Danny de Vries

Definition	• Balloon expandable stent • Slotted tube • Multiple cells with multiple 'V' connectors

History	• 1998 Design • 1998 First clinical experience • 1999 CE approval • 1999 Clinical use in Europe

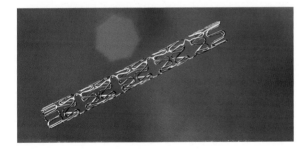

Figure 25.1: *Stent unmounted un-expanded. The Nexus stent is a balloon expandable stent. It has a tubular design, with multiple cells and multiple 'V' connections for high radial strength combined with longitudinal flexibility. It is available unmounted and premounted on a rapid exchange balloon.*

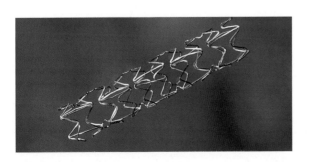

Figure 25.2: *Expanded stent.*

Tips and tricks for delivery

This sheathless rapid exchange premounted Nexus stent needs little preparation time. Prior to introduction negative pressure is applied to the catheter and seating of stent checked with rinsed gloves.

Primary stenting is often possible owing to the low profile and high flexibility of the Nexus stent. Placement of the stent in bifurcation and in ostial lesions and subsequent treatment of side branches, including stenting through the struts, is possible.

Full deployment of the Nexus stent is at < 6 atm.

Indications for use

- Dissection
- Tortuous vessels
- Bifurcations
- Small vessels
- Bail out
- Bypass grafts
- Distal vessels
- Long lesions
- Suboptimal PTCA
- Adjunct to other devices

Nexus stent technical specifications

Material composition:	316 LVM Stainless steel
Degree of radiopacity (grade):	Moderate
Ferromagnetism:	Non-ferromagnetic (MRI safe)
Metallic surface area (expanded):	13.6% at 3.0 mm diameter
Metallic cross-sectional area:	0.182 mm^2
Stent design:	Laser cut from a stainless steel tube
Strut dimensions:	0.0047 inch (0.120 mm) thick 0.0041 inch (0.105 mm) wide
Delivery profile (crossing profile):	0.9–1.0 mm
Longitudinal flexibility:	High
Percentage shortening on expansion:	2.6% (3.0 mm stent)
Expansion range:	2.5–5.0 mm
Degree of recoil (shape memory):	2% (3 mm stent)
Radial force (to collapse):	1690 Mn average
Currently available diameters:	2.5–5.0 mm unmounted
Currently available lengths:	8, 12, 15, 18, 23 and 28 mm
Currently available diameters:	2.5–5.0 mm mounted
Recrossability of implanted stents:	Very good
Available bare (unmounted):	Yes
Other coronary types available:	None

Nexus stent delivery system

Mechanism of deployment:	Balloon expandable
Catheter type:	Rapid exchange
Shaft profile:	2.0
Guidewire compatibility:	0.014 inch (0.36 mm)
Minimal internal diameter of guiding catheter:	0.064 inch (1.6 mm), 6 Fr
Balloon material:	Semi compliant gamma radiation modified copolymer
Balloon diameters:	2.5, 3.0, 3.5 and 4.0 mm
Position of radiopaque markers:	Proximal and distal to stent
Rated burst pressure of balloon:	14 Atm

Why I like my stent

- Rapid exchange system
- Low profile
- High flexibility
- Excellent conformability
- Moderate radiopacity
- Optimal radial strength
- Sheathless deployment system
- Suitable for a wide range of applications
- Easy side branch access

Case example

The following is a case treated with the Nexus stent (Muenchen–Bogenhausen in April 1999 by Prof. Thomas Ischinger). A diffuse lesion in the LAD (Figure 25.3) was treated by using one 2.5 × 18 mm Nexus stent leaving a good result with the stent following the natural curvature of the vessel while preserving its sidebranch (Figure 25.4).

Figure 25.5 shows the position and radiopacity of the Nexus stent after deployment.

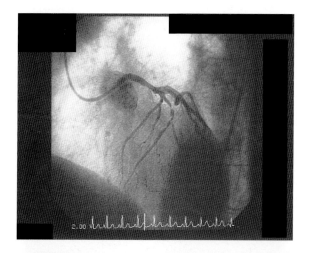

Figure 25.3:
Diffuse lesion in LAD.

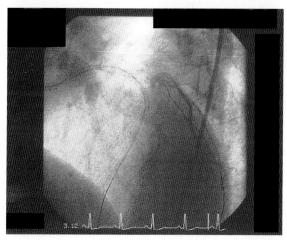

Figure 25.4:
Post-stenting, adapting the natural curvature of the vessel.

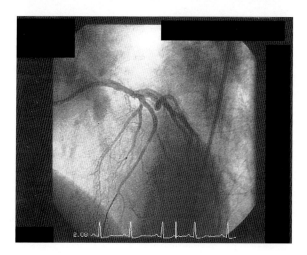

Figure 25.5:
Control angiogram.

Clinical experience

During the initial clinical tests, 99% of all placements were successful 40% in the LAD, 32% in the RCA, 12% in the Diagonal, 4% in the LCX and 12% in Bypass Grafts. Of these, 40% were used for primary stenting without predilatation.

Deployment pressure ranged from 6 to 14 atm with a median of 10 atm. A multicenter European registry is currently underway.

Nexus II stent technical specifications

Material composition:	316 LVM stainless steel
Degree of radiopacity (grade):	Good
Ferromagnetism:	Non-ferromagnetic (MRI safe)
Metallic surface area expanded:	18.9% at 3 mm diameter
Metallic cross-sectional area:	0.182 mm²
Stent design:	Laser cut from a stainless steel tube
Strut dimensions:	0.0047 inch (0.120 mm) thick 0.0041 inch (0.105 mm) thick
Delivery profile(crossing profile):	0.9–1.0 mm
Longitudinal flexibility:	Very good
Percentage shortening (on delivery):	N/a
Percentage shortening on expansion:	1.67% avg (3 mm stent)
Expansion range:	2.5–5.0 mm
Degree of recoil (shape memory):	2.74% for a 3 mm stent
Radial force (to collapse):	Excellent 2394 Mn avg
Currently available diameters:	2.5–5.0 mm unmounted
Currently available lengths:	8, 12, 15, 18 and 23 mm
Currently available diameters:	2.5–5.0 mm mounted
Recrossability of implanted stent:	Very good
Available bare (unmounted):	Yes

Nexus II stent delivery system

Mechanism of deployment:	Balloon expandable
Catheter type:	Rapid exchange
Shaft profile:	2.0 Fr
Guidewire compatibility:	0.014 inch (0.36 mm)
Minimal internal diameter of guiding catheter:	0.064 inch (1.6 mm)
Balloon material:	Semi-compliant, gamma radiation modified copolymer
Balloon diameters:	2.5, 3.0, 3.5 and 4.0 mm
Position of radiopaque markers:	Proximal and distal to stent
Rated burst pressure of balloon:	16 atm

Why I like my stent

- Very flexible
- Low profile
- Excellent side branch access
- Conforms well to balloon in angled vessels
- Smooth vessel appearance post-stenting
- Easy stent through stent
- Dilatable cells
- Visibility
- Minimal recoil

Case example

The following is a case treated with the Nexus II stent (Muenchen–Bogenhausen performed by Professor Thomas Ischinger). A 63-year-old male with unstable angina, double vessel CAD (100% RCA with collaterals, 80% left circumflex artery) and bilateral internal carotid artery stenosis of 90%. The interventional strategy was to correct the RCA first and then, during a second session, the bilateral ICA problem.

205

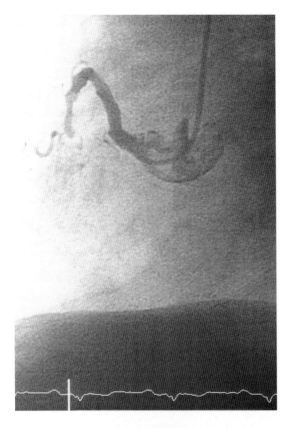

Figure 25.6: *Total proximal occlusion of RCA with difficult anatomy (shepherd's hook configuration). The procedure was performed using a 5 Fr (Medtronic) AL2 guiding catheter and a 0.014 inch Galeo (Biotronik) wire and balloons (NERO) and stents (NEXUS II) from OCCAM International. Routine medical Tx (heparin, ASS, clopidogrel) and bolus of integrilin.*

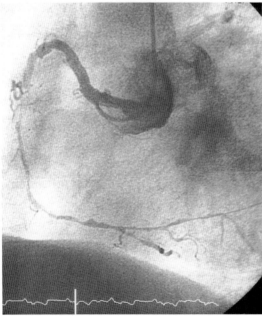

Figure 25.7: *Partial recanalization, severely diseased artery.*

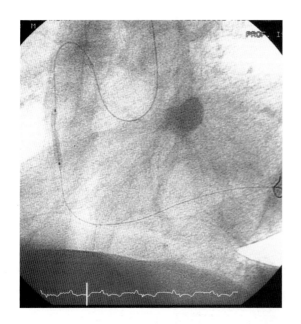

Figure 25.8: *Multiple dilatations with 2.5 and 3.0 balloons (Nero, OCCAM).*

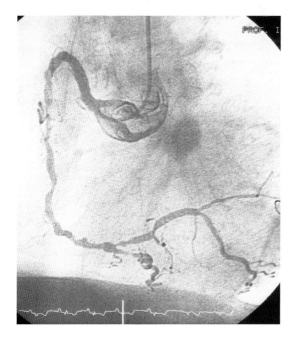

Figure 25.9: *RCA prior to stent implantations. Suspicion of thrombus in proximal segment.*

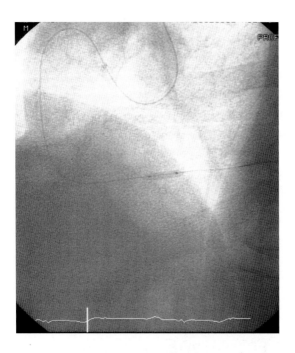

Figure 25.10: *Placement of very distal stent (NEXUS II, 2.5 × 12 mm).*

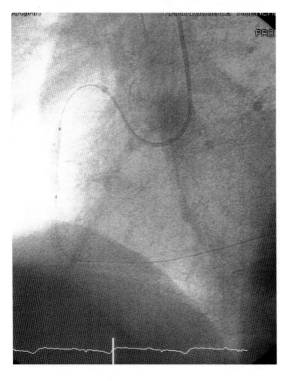

Figure 25.11: *Placement of one of the more proximal stents (NEXUS II, 3.5 × 18 mm).*

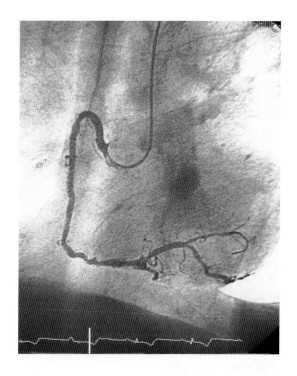

Figure 25.12: *After placement of four stents with one moderately (untreated) stenotic segment distally.*

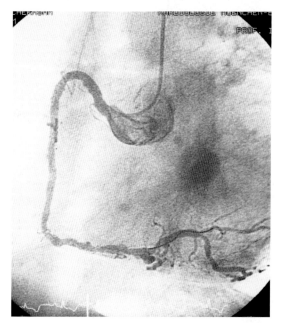

Figure 25.13: *After final distal dilatation with moderate residual stenosis.*

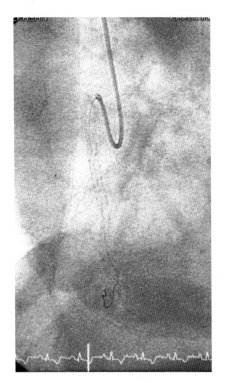

Figure 25.14

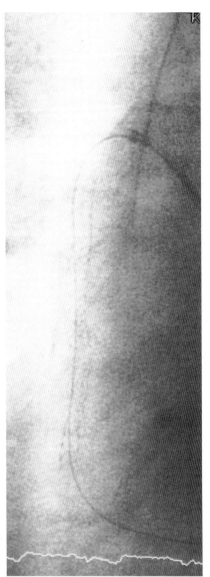

Figure 25.15

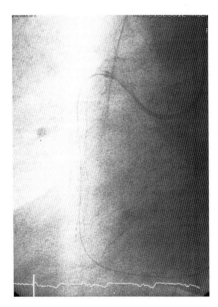

Figure 25.16

Figures 25.14–25.16: Balanced radiopacity of the NEXUS II Stent.

Comment

This case illustrates multiple stenting in a severely diseased and recanalized artery with challenging anatomy, using a 5 French guiding catheter. A total of four stents were placed (2.5 × 8 mm, 3.0 × 15 mm, 3.5 × 18 mm and 3.5 × 12 mm). The Nexus II stent comes in all routinely usable lengths, 8 mm to 28 mm), is very flexible and moderately radiopaque. In this case, the challenge was to pass multiple NEXUS stents through very tortuous anatomy (including passage through a NEXUS stent) and a diffusely diseased artery. In particular, flexibility, safe fixation of the stent on the balloon and visibility of the stent for precise positioning were the most important qualities. The low profile and smoothness of the NEXUS II permits use of 5 Fr guiding systems, even for large (> 3 mm) stent sizes. The design permits easy side branch access. The stents were placed with pressures from 9 atm (distal stent) to 15 atm.

Clinical experience

During the initial clinical tests, Nexus II stent delivery systems were implanted by seven physicians with a 100% success rate.

In 54% direct stenting was performed. The rest had prior PTCA or sub-optimal results needing stent placement.

The majority used 6 Fr guiding catheters, in 18% a 5 Fr guiding catheter was used. Residual stenosis during implantation was below 3.5%. The stent delivery pressure used ranged from 10 to 14 atm.

Fifty per cent of stents were placed in the right coronary artery, 36% in the left coronary and 14% in bypass grafts.

Currently over 1500 units have been implanted worldwide.

26. THE NIR AND NIRFLEX CORONARY STENTS

Medinol Ltd, Tel Aviv, Israel

Kobi Richter, Yaron Almagor and Martin Leon

Description

General

The NIR Stent was developed based on many physicians' 'wish list' for new functional features in order to overcome shortcomings of first generation devices. The two most important features of the coronary stent are basic to its use: the radial force with which it supports the vessel, and its flexibility, one of the major determinants of its trackability into the target lesion before deployment. The basic contradiction between flexible structure that enable good trackability and rigid structure that result in optimal support, brought the developers of first generation stents to select one property while compromising on the other. A typical comparison of features resulting from that forced decision is:

Stent	Radial support	Flexibility
Palmaz–Schatz	High	Low
Gianturco–Roubin	Low	High

Our primary goal in designing the NIR Stent was to overcome this compromise by a new design for the stent, with a secondary goal to optimize other clinically important features.

Transforming geometry

A design goal was defined noticing that the two features are not required simultaneously, but rather at two mutually exclusive time slices.

* Flexibility is required only during insertion and until deployment of the stent at the target lesion.
* Rigidity is required to supply long term support to the vessel wall only from the moment of deployment and on.

It was thus defined that the desired geometry should be flexible upon insertion and will change after deployment to be rigid upon expansion.

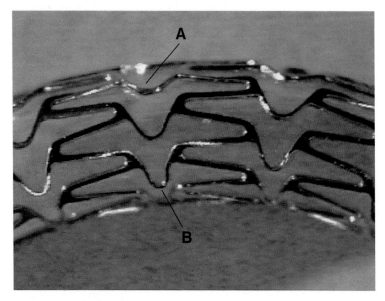

Figure 26.1: *The NIR stent before expansion, showing the differentially elongating cells. The cell inside the curve is shorter than its counterpart outside the curve, as shown by the converging lines at their border. This feature is enabled by the vertical loop component of the cell that opens on the outside cell (A) and closes on the inside cell (B).*

Trackability and flexibility

The flexibility of a stent, a long stent especially, is a major parameter in determining its trackability into the naturally curved and tortuous anatomy of diseased coronary arteries. In order to track into such anatomies the stent on its delivery system has to curve around corners or it will latch on the opposing vessel wall. The flexibility depends on the ability of the stent to elongate differentially such that the stent wall outside of the curve be longer than the wall inside the curve. Inability or high resistance to such differential elongation will not allow the stent to flex. The design of the NIR stent is based on uniform cells each of which is capable of elongating or foreshortening as demonstrated in Figure 26.1.

Other important features that facilitate the trackability of the stent are:

1. The stent has no 'free internal points' loops or ends internal to the tubular structure that are not connected longitudinally to their neighbors and thus can flare out and generate internal ridges that will latch on plaque surface upon insertion (Figure 26.2).
2. The stent has a very low profile and crimps easily and securely on the balloon

owing to the original structure with struts slightly open (see Figure 26.1) that leaves a lot of room for crimping until struts touch each other (see Figure 26.2).

3. Most of the struts are along the insertion direction of the stent and thus will not catch on plaque the way a typical coiled stent would (see Figure 26.2).

NIR stent technical specifications

Material composition:	Stainless steel
Degree of radiopacity:	Moderate
Ferromagnetism:	Nonferromagnetic (MRI safe)
Metallic surface area (metal: artery, expanded):	11–18%
Degree of recoil (shape memory):	<1%
Strut design:	Square, transform from flexible to rigid
Strut thickness:	0.004 inch (0.1 mm)
Non-expanded profile:	<0.04 inch (<1.0 mm)
Longitudinal flexibility:	High upon insertion, low after expansion
Percentage shortening on expansion:	<3%
Currently available diameters:	2–5 mm
Currently available lengths:	9, 16, 25 and 32 mm
Other non-coronary types:	Peripheral stents for peripheral vessels, biliary, renal and other uses: lengths: 14, 19, 39 and 59 mm. Expanded diameter range: 5–12 mm

NIR stent delivery system

Mechanism of deployment:	Balloon expandable
Minimal internal diameter of guiding catheter:	0.064 inch (1.6 mm), 6Fr
Premounted on delivery catheter:	Yes
Available bare (unmounted):	Yes
Protective sheath/cover:	No
Position of radiopaque markers:	Proximal and distal to stent
Further balloon expansion recommended:	No
Recrossability of implanted stents:	Excellent
Sizing diameter:	Matching target vessel diameter

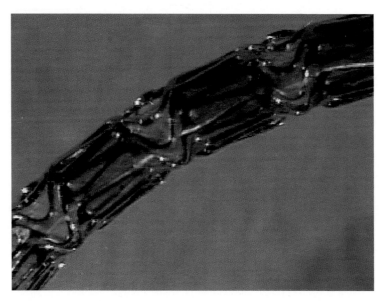

Figure 26.2: *The crimped NIR stent, showing a low profile of less than 1.0 mm and a smooth surface with no internal flare-out points at the outside of a curved section. Notice also the difference between the slightly open struts of Figure 26.1 and the tightly crimped struts at this figure.*

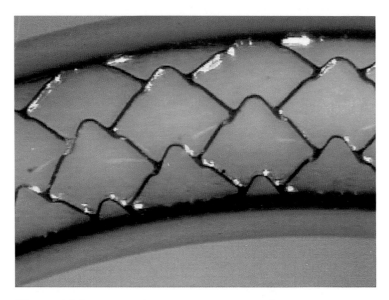

Figure 26.3: *The expanded NIR stent, showing uniform cells in which the vertical loop struts have aligned with the horizontal loop struts to form straight struts. The resulting structure is a very rigid and strong structure.*

Rigidity and radial support

During expansion of the stent in the target lesion the geometry of the basic uniform cell changes (Figure 26.3) in a way that will cause the vertical loops of the cell to align with the horizontal loops and form a diamond-like cell with straight struts at about 45°.

The resulting diamond-like mesh with interlinked struts is much stronger and more rigid than any structure without such interlinking. At this point in time the stent loses its flexibility, but this lost feature is no longer important since the stent is not required to move anywhere.

Important features of the expanded NIR stent

1. The uniform cellular design allows for a continuous support without gaps unlike articulations in other stents, or increased distance between struts that may occur in stents whose struts are not interlinked and move relative to each other.

2. The relatively small cells decreased the chance for tissue prolapse and plaque scale protrusion into the lumen. The smaller cells made of shorter struts provide for higher radial resistance and decreased wall trauma by decreasing the local pressure on the wall. The number of circumferential struts in the NIR stent is 18 and in the Palmaz–Schatz 8, thus at an equal total radial force the local force applied by each strut is less than one half in the NIR stent.

3. The differential elongation of the vertical loops of the cells, responsible for the flexibility upon insertion, allows for conformance of the stent with the vessel curvature such that the rigid expanded stent does not straighten the vessel and does not create a sharp kink at the interface between the stented area and the unstented area. Such a kink created by other rigid stents (e.g. Palmaz–Schatz may cause turbulence and applies excessive local pressure that accounts for a higher restenosis rate at the stent ends. That feature of conformance with vessel curvature (see Figure 26.3) allows also for multiple stenting of long segments required in many cases of diffuse disease and generates a smooth conformed reconstructed section.

4. Most stents available on the market foreshorten upon expansion by varied amounts owing to the change in diameter of the stent. The combination of vertical loops and horizontal loops in the NIR cell results in minimized foreshortening based on the fact that upon expansion the horizontal loops foreshorten but the vertical loops elongate and compensate for the foreshortening thus keeping the total length of the cell unchanged (Figure 26.4).

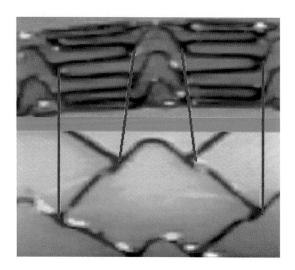

Figure 26.4: *While the cell expands the horizontal loops foreshorten and the vertical loops elongate to leave the total length of the cell unchanged.*

Case example

The following is an example of a case treated with the NIR stent. It is from the first pilot study performed in the Centro Cuore in Milan on July 1995, by Drs Colombo, Almagor and DiMario.

Case 1:

A 32-mm stent was inserted into a very tortuous RCA using a right Judkins guiding catheter. In spite of the suboptimal support the stent tracked into the vessel smoothly to yield a good result in a very short procedure involving a single stent.

Conclusion

The NIR stent is a second generation stent with improved functional features, as demonstrated by its geometry clinical results.

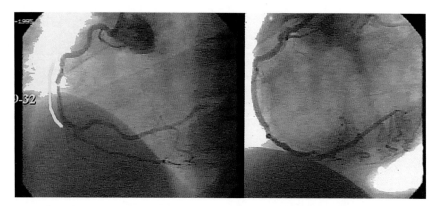

Figure 26.5: *A 32-mm NIR stent was inserted into a very tortuous RCA, demonstrating the trackability of the stent. The result on the right would require at least two stents of other designs.*

218

NIROYAL™ stent technical specifications

Material composition:	Stainless steel plated with gold
Degree of radiopacity:	Excellent
Ferromagnetism:	Nonferromagnetic (MRI safe)
Metallic surface area (metal: artery, expanded):	11–18%
Degree of recoil:	<0.5%
Strut design:	Rounded square, transforms from flexible to rigid upon expansion
Strut thickness:	0.004 inch (0.1 mm)
Non-expanded profile:	0.04 inch (< 1.0 mm)
Longitudinal flexibility:	Excellent upon insertion, reduced after expansion
Percentage shortening on expansion:	<3%
Currently available diameter:	2–5 mm
Currently available lengths:	9, 16, 25, 32 mm
Other non-coronary types:	Peripheral stents length: 14, 19, 39, 59 mm, diameter 5–12 mm

New features available

Two main new features have been introduced to the coronary market since the first edition. A pre-mounted system and the NIROYAL gold plated radiopaque stent. The pre-mounted system, the NIR PRIMO™, features the NIR™ PRIMO™ stent pre-mounted on a modified VIVA PRIMO™ balloon catheter from SciMED. The pre-mounted system saves time as crimping is not required and increases safety by a better and more consistent crimping. The system also features a short ring of plastic material inserted under the balloon in front of the stent. This increases the diameter of the balloon in front of the stent and creates a 'dam' that prevents the stent from slipping off the balloon (see Figure 26.6).

The NIROYAL stent is a NIR stent plated with gold (see Figure 26.7) to increase its radiopacity. The stent has indeed a drastically improved radiopacity (see Figure 26.8) that allows its visualization before and after expansion. The radiopacity of the NIROYAL was, nevertheless, designed such that the stent will be visible but will not hide angiographic details after its deployment (see Figures 26.9–26.16). The radiopacity of the NIROYAL is important for positioning judgment by the physician, and especially in cases of multiple stents for judgment of overlap, and in bifurcation and ostial stenting where relative position is critical.

219

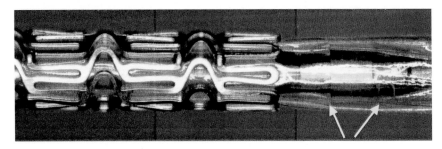

Figure 26.6: *The distal tip of the stent premounted on a balloon, showing the 'Dam' (arrows).*

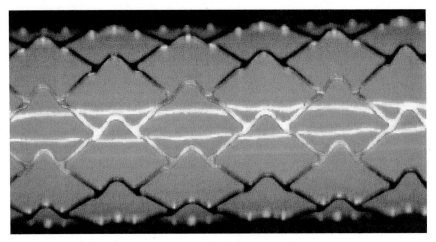

Figure 26.7: *The NIROYAL stent after expansion.*

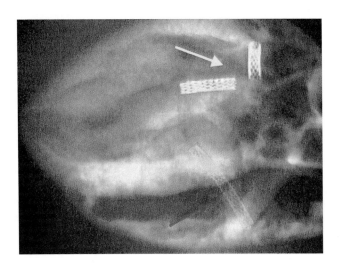

Figure 26.8:
An X-ray radiograph of an excised porcine heart shows the excellent radiopacity of the NIROYAL stents (yellow arrow), as compared to the regular NIR stent (red arrow).

Case example

The following is an example of a case treated with new NIR stents. It is a case of a bifurcation stenting performed with the NIROYAL.

Case 1:

A lesion in the LAD involving an ostial lesion in the first diagonal was selected for treatment (Figure 26.9). A 32 mm long NIROYAL was placed in the LAD across the bifurcation of the diagonal (Figures 26.10 and 26.11). A second, 9 mm long NIROYAL was inserted into the diagonal through the cells of the LAD stent (Figures 26.12 and 26.13). The diagonal stent left a gap at the ostium uncovered (Figure 26.14) and a third NIROYAL was placed to bridge the gap (Figure 26.15) to yield a good final result (Figure 26.16).

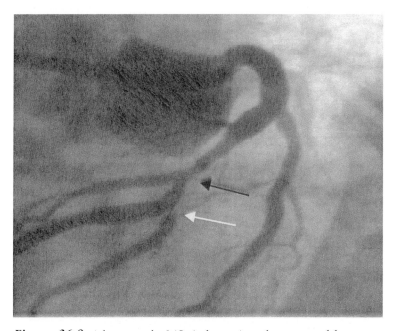

Figure 26.9: *A lesion in the LAD (red arrow) overlaps an ostial lesion in the diagonal (yellow arrow).*

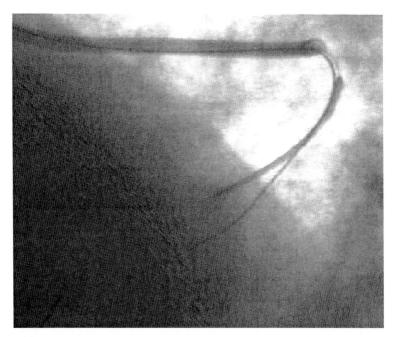

Figure 26.10: *The 32 mm NIROYAL is placed in the LAD showing its radiopacity.*

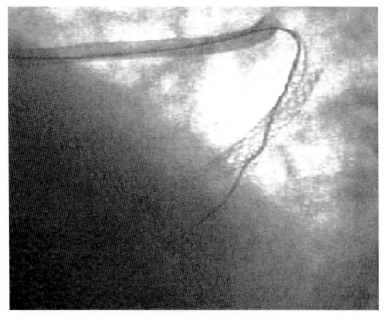

Figure 26.11: *The NIROYAL expanded in the LAD.*

222

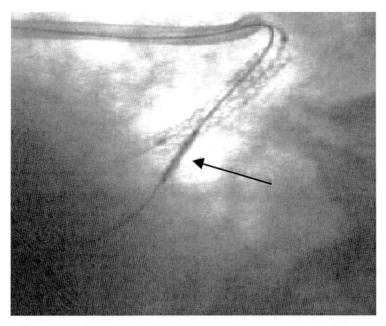

Figure 26.12: *The short NIROYAL (arrow) is placed in the diagonal through the struts of the expanded stent.*

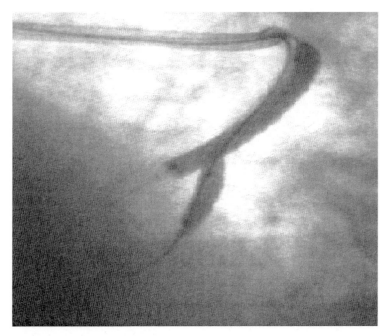

Figure 26.13: *The second stent is deployed using 'kissing balloons' technique.*

223

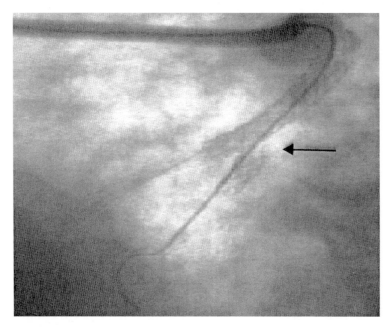

Figure 26.14: *The two expanded stents show a gap (arrow) at the ostium of the diagonal.*

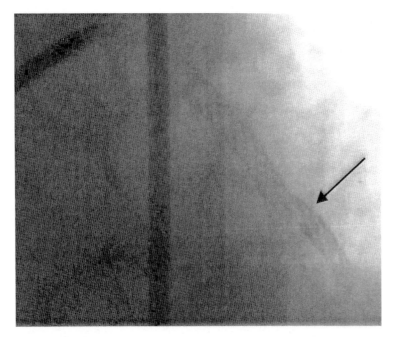

Figure 26.15: *After deployment of a third stent (arrow) the bifurcation is fully covered.*

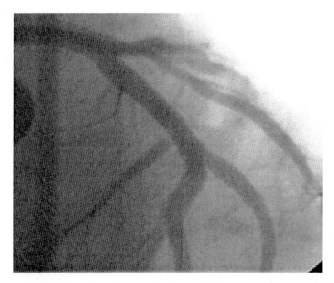

Figure 26.16: *Final result demonstrating that the NIROYAL does not hide angiographic details.*

New NIR® Stent Family Features

Several new NIR® products were introduced to the coronary stent market during the year 2000. The NIROYAL™ Advance, NIR® Elite and NIROYAL™ Elite pre-mounted stent systems were launched on the Monorail platform while the NIR® w/SOX stent system was launched on the OTW platform. Each of these products included one or more of the new stent technologies offered by Boston Scientific/Scimed, namely the NIROYAL™ stent, the conformer NIR® stent design, and the SOX™ system technology.

NIROYAL™ Stent

The NIROYAL™ Stent is a gold-plated NIR® stent, providing increased radiopacity. The drastically improved radiopacity of the NIROYAL™ stent allows improved visualization of the stent before and after expansion. The radiopacity of the NIROYAL™ was designed such that the stent would be visible but would not hide angiographic details after its deployment. The radiopacity of the NIROYAL™ is important for accurate stent placement (e.g. multiple stents, side branch positioning, and full lesion coverage) and precise post dilatation. The increased positioning accuracy is very important when the stent elutes anti-proliferative drug and the drug concentration relative to the treated lesion is critical.

225

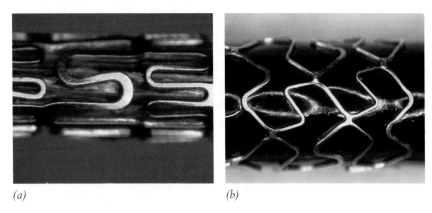

(a)   (b)

Figure 26.17: *The NIRFLEX before expansion (a) on the left demonstrates a smooth structure with struts mainly along the insertion axis. After expansion (b) the closed cells have each three "Compartments" each of which is smaller than the whole cell resulting in a more continuous coverage than even the original NIR stent.*

NIR® Stent with Conformer Design

The NIR® and NIROYAL™ Stents with Conformer Design have recently been introduced. This design incorporates a NIR® Stent geometry with modified end cells and shorter end struts. The aim of this design is to minimize stent edge flaring, allow improved trackability, and provide improved vessel conformability and increased radial strength at the stent ends. In recent trials in pigs, long stents with this configuration showed lower restenosis due to less tension induced in the vessel wall.

NIRFLEX™

The NIRFLEX stent, which is the new stent design of Medinol, started a pilot trial in 2000 and was completed in 2001. The stent will start a worldwide multicenter randomized trial with long-term angiographic follow up in 2001. The NIRFLEX is a unique design that combines for the first time a flexibility before and after deployment that is second to no stent, with the continuous coverage of vessel wall so typical of the NIR family of stents. The stent was tried in pigs and showed very low restenosis rate with long stents, typical of its continuous coverage and excellent conformability. The stent will be tried and later released as a stainless steel (SST) stent and also gold plated but with gold that undergoes a special thermal treatment that smoothes it and seals it which results in a restenosis rate identical to that of SST stent of the same design. The continuous coverage and the uniform strut density inside and outside a curved stented section of a vessel makes this stent the ideal choice for drug coating as it potentially results in uniform drug concentrations in the underlying tissue, the importance of which has been recently demonstrated in scientific trials. Images of the NIRFLEX before and after expansion are shown in Figure 26.17.

References

1. Almagor Y, Feld S, Kiemeneij F et al, for the FINESS Trial Investigators. First international new intravascular rigid-flex endovascular stent study (FINESS): clinical and angiographic results after elective and urgent stent implantation. *J Am Coll Cardiol* 1997;**30**:847–54.

2. Almagor Y, Feld S, Kiemeneij F et al. First international new intravascular rigid-flex endovascular stent study: angiographic results and six month clinical follow-up. *Eur Heart J* 1997;**18**(suppl):156.

3. Di Mario C, Reimers B, Almagor Y et al. Procedural and follow-up results with a new balloon expandable stent in unselected lesions. *Heart* 1998;**79**:234–41.

4. Zheng H, Corcos T, Favereau X, Pentousis D, Guérin Y, Ouzan J. Preliminary experience with the NIR coronary stent. *Catheter Cardiovasc Diagn* 1998;**43**:153–58.

5. Lau KW, He Q, Ding ZP, Quek S, Johan A. Early experience with the NIR intracoronary stent. *Am J Cardiol* 1998;**81**:927–29.

6. Chevalier B, Lefevre T, Meyer P et al. French registry of seven cells NIRstent implantation in ≤2.5 mm coronary arteries [abstract]. *Circulation* 1997;**96**(suppl):I-274.

7. Lansky AJ, Popma JJ, Mehran R et al. Late quantitative angiographic results after NIR stent use: results from the NIRVANA randomized trial and registries [abstract]. *J Am Coll Cardiol* 1998;**31**(suupl):80A.

8. Baim DS. Acute and 30-day clinical results of the NIRVANA Trial [abstract]. *Circulation* 1997;**96**(suppl):I-594.

27. THE PROLINK STENT

Vascular Concepts Limited, Crawley, UK

Thomas A Ischinger

Description	• Balloon expandable stent • Corrugated ultrathin ring design • Thin rings interconnected by three alternating links • Stent mounted on low profile balloon • Extremely low profile (3.0 mm stent has a profile of 0.039 inch) • Excellent side-branch access • Minimal foreshortening on expansion • Wall thickness of 0.0028 mm provides optimum radial strength • Initial deployment pressure 5 atm • Available premounted on a rapid exchange balloon catheter with 1.8 Fr • Shaft and a high pressure compliant balloon

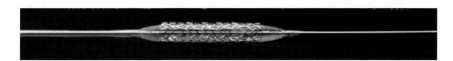

Figure 27.1: Expansion of the Prolink stent shows even expansion throughout the length of the stent.

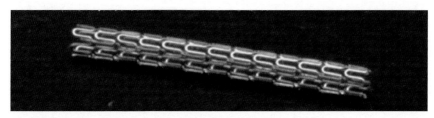

Figure 27.2: Unexpanded Prolink stent with its 'thin wall' design.

Prolink stent technical specifications

Material composition:	316 L stainless steel
Degree of radiopacity:	Moderate
Ferromagnetism:	Non-ferromagnetic (MRI safe)
Metallic surface area: (metal: artery expanded)	Less than 15%
Stent design:	Laser cut from stainless steel tube in a ring pattern, ring interconnected by three alternating links.
Strut dimensions:	0.0028 mm wall, 0.0028 mm strut width
Longitudinal flexibility:	High
Foreshortening:	Less than 2%
Profile on delivery system:	Less than 3 Fr
Radial force:	Moderate
Degree of recoil:	Minimal
Side branch access:	Excellent
Available diameters:	2.5–4.0 mm
Available lengths:	10, 15, 20, 25, 30 mm
Recrossability:	Excellent

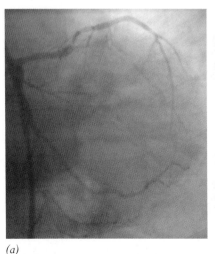 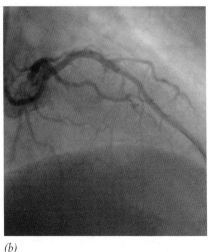

(a)   (b)

Figure 27.3: Before (a) implantation of the Prolink stent in a tight tortuous lesion and subsequently after (b) implantation. NOTE: Conformability of the stent to the tortuous lesion.

230

Prolink combo stent delivery system

Mechanism of deployment:	Balloon expandable
Minimal recommended guiding catheter:	6 Fr
Balloon types:	Rapid exchange
Balloon characteristics:	High pressure, semicompliant
Balloon material:	Polyamide co-blend
Offered as a bare stent:	Yes
Protective sheath:	No
Balloon compliance:	Nominal at 6, 10% compliance after 6 atm
Rated burst pressure of the balloon:	19 atm
Delivery profile:	2.5 mm–0.037 mm 3.0 mm–0.038 mm 3.5 mm–0.039 mm
Longitudinal flexibility:	High
Stent retention:	High
Sizing diameter:	2.5, 3.0 and 3.5 mm
Recrossability of implanted stent:	Good

Indications for clinical use

- Direct stenting
- Tortuous anatomy
- Restenotic lesions
- Lesions on a bend
- Side branch placement
- Acute closure and bailout
- Totally occluded artery
- De novo lesions
- Acute MI
- Suboptimal PTCA

Why I like my stent

The Prolink stent is a fully closed cell design mounted on a low profile delivery system and provides clinicians with the most preferred attributes in a stent:

1. Flexibility and extremely low profile enables direct stenting
2. Optimal radial strength, provides good conformability to the vessel wall
3. No plaque prolapse at the implanted sites
4. 19 atm rated burst pressure stent delivery system
5. 6 Fr guide compatibility
6. Able to cross 99% occluded vessels

The clinical performance with the Prolink stent has been superior and comparable to any of the existing coronary stent systems. FEM and other analysis have validated the mechanical properties and its 'thin wall design'.

28. THE PROPASS STENT
(Platinum activated stent surface)

Vascular Concepts Limited, Crawley, UK

Thomas A Ischinger

Vascular Concepts has developed the first ever platinum activated stent. The rationale behind the platinum coating was to coat the base stainless steel surface with a more biocompatible, inert material that illicts a lower tissue reaction and injury upon implantation in the vessel. The objective was also to increase the radiopacity of the base stent by using a microthin platinum which provides uniform visibility before and after implantation.

Coating methodology

The ProPass is coated with a thin film of platinum-iridium, which renders the surface antithrombogenic and enhances biocompatibility compared to the bare stainless steel. The platinum coating is deposited using the ion deposition process where an atomic layer of platinum is first deposited followed by a secondary layer of atoms. Platinum–iridium has been used for the last two decades in pacemaker leads. It has very unique physical and chemical characteristics: inertness, low weight, scratch resistance, elasticity, strength, softness and wear resistance. The coating is performed in a high vacuum atmosphere on a proprietary planetary fixture that involves coating both on the inside and the outside of the stent in a uniform pattern. X-ray diffraction analysis has shown that the outside and the inside surface of the stent is covered only with platinum, iridium and the nickel, iron, chromium of the base stainless steel is completely covered.

Preclinical animal studies

Preliminary animal studies conducted at the Skejby University in Aarhus, Denmark have demonstrated that over a 30-day period, there was no adverse reactions to the stent implantations. No subacute problems were recorded and the intimal growth at the end of 30 days was less than 8%.
A more detailed 90-day preclinical study is currently underway at the Armed Forces Institute of Pathology, Washington DC.

Clinical investigation

An initial multicentre registry trial of 125 patients has been completed in India. Follow-up of these patients has shown a 0% subacute thrombosis rate and no major clinical events to date.

A multicenter study comparing the ProPass (Platinum Activated Stent Surface) with the Prolink is currently underway in Europe and preliminary results are anticipated by the end of 2001.

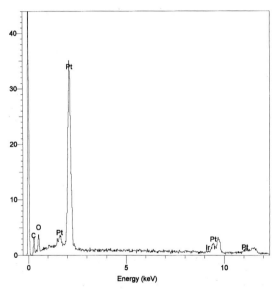

Figure 28.1: EDAX Analysis of the inside surface of the ProPass stent shows absence of nickel/iron/chromium on the surface of the stent.

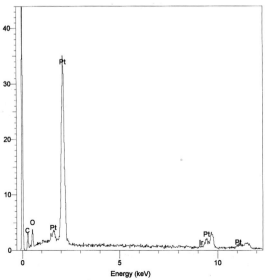

Figure 28.2: EDAX Analysis of the outside surface of the ProPass stent shows absence of nickel/iron/chromium on the surface of the stent.

ProPass stent technical specifications

Material composition:	Base 316 L stainless steel
Degree of radiopacity:	Moderate
Ferromagnetism:	Non-ferromagnetic (MRI safe)
Metallic surface area: (metal: artery expanded)	Less than 15%
Stent design:	Laser cut from stainless steel tube in a ring pattern, ring interconnected by three alternating links.
Strut dimensions:	0.0028 mm wall, 0.0028 mm strut width
Longitudinal flexibility:	High
Foreshortening:	Less than 2%
Profile on delivery system:	Less than 3 Fr
Radial force:	Moderate
Degree of recoil:	Minimal
Side branch access:	Excellent
Available diameters:	2.5–4.0 mm
Available lengths:	10, 15, 20, 25, 30 mm
Recrossability:	Excellent

ProPass stent delivery system

Mechanism of deployment:	Balloon expandable
Protective sheath:	No
Design:	Rapid exchange
Balloon characteristics:	Semi-compliant
Rated burst pressure:	19 atm
Recommended deployment pressure:	12 atm
Guidewire compatibility:	0.014 inch
Minimal internal diameter of guide catheter:	6 Fr
Offered as a bare stent:	Yes

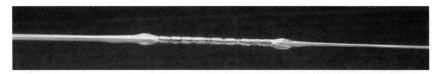

Figure 28.3: *Low profile balloon-mounted ProPass stent system.*

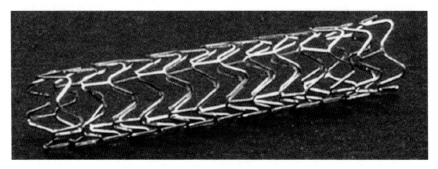

Figure 28.4: *A fully expanded mounted ProPass stent.*

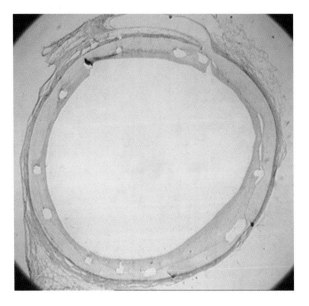

Figure 28.5:
Histopathologic cross-section of a pig coronary artery 28 days after implantation of the ProPass stent.

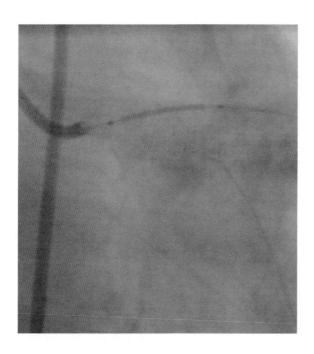

Figure 28.6:
Radiopacity of the ProPass stent facilitates precise positioning in the lesion.

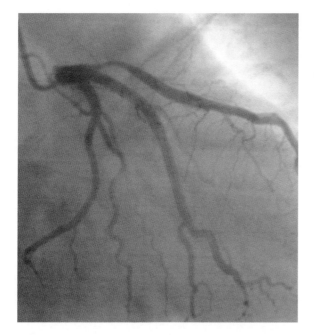

Figure 28.7: *A tight ostial lesion requires good positioning flexibility and conformability.*

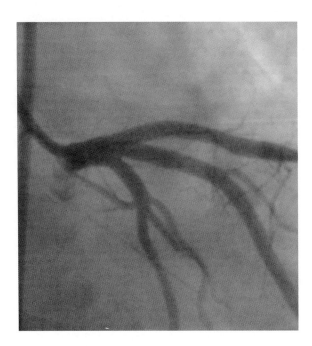

Figure 28.8: *ProPass stent implanted in the lesion in Figure 28.7.*

29. THE CORONARY R STENT™

Orbus Medical Technologies, Inc, Fort Lauderdale, FL, USA

David P Foley, H Richard Davis and Jurgen Ligthart

Description

The R Stent is composed of three distinct zones. The end zones located at
the extremities of the stent anchor the entire structure during deployment
and provide squared ends rather than the obliquely oriented leading and
trailing margins of coil stents which may lead to imprecise positioning and
uneven or imperfect support. The center zone of the R Stent consists of a
continuous dual helix lattice. In between the end and center zones is a
transition zone which mates the dual helix lattice to the ends of the stent.
This configuration provides the R stent with omni-directional flexibility,
extremely high radial strength, and optimal side branch access.

The R Stent is made from medical grade 316 L stainless steel, which has
a well-characterized bio-safety profile as an implant material. The strut
thickness of the R-Stent allows for reasonable radiopacity without
obscuring the lesion area.

Although it was the practice in most centers to predilate all coronary
lesions before stent implantation, during the last few years direct coronary
stenting without predilatation has been quickly developing as the new
therapeutic approach with both a potential healthcare as well as health-
economic benefit. The R Stent on the EVOLUTION is a low profile, semi-
compliant Rapid Exchange PTCA dilatation catheter which facilitates direct
stenting. The stent is well matched to this catheter with 0.5 mm of the
balloon exposed on the leading and trailing edges. The system has a
nominal deployment pressure of 10 atm and at the rated burst pressure of
16 atm, which is capable of increasing the stent 0.25 mm beyond its
nominal diameter. The stent is mounted to the balloon between two
radiopaque marker bands that delimit the working length of the balloon. In
addition, the delivery system also has two (2) markers on the trailing shaft,
which indicate the exit of the delivery system tip from the guiding
catheter. These attributes combined with a robust crimping process and the
resulting excellent crossing profile allow access in most coronary artery
lesions without predilatation.

History	1997	First human implants, Thoraxcenter, Erasmus University Medical Centre Rotterdam, The Netherlands
	1998	Completion of the first clinical feasibility study at the Thoraxcenter, Erasmus University Medical Centre Rotterdam, The Netherlands Orbus is ISO9001 certified
	1999	CE Mark for the Coronary R Stent. R Stent in mounted on the Talos SDS and approved for sale in Europe
	2000	Initiation of the first multicenter registry – RESTOR Initiation of the first multicenter randomized study – DIRECTOR
	2001	Product launch of the R Stent mounted on the EVOLUTION SDS

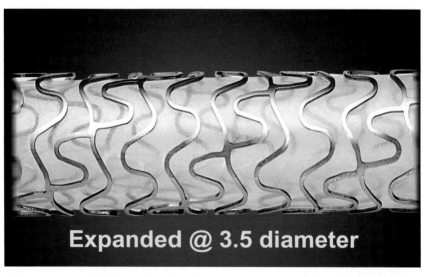

Expanded @ 3.5 diameter

Figure 29.1: Picture of a loose stent.

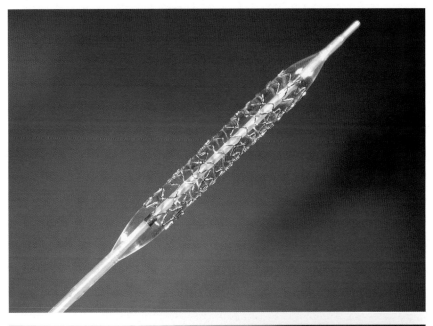

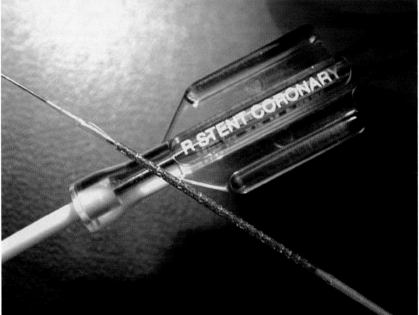

Figure 29.2: *Picture of stent and delivery system.*

241

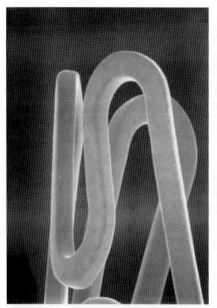
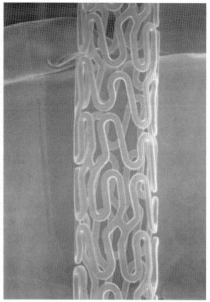
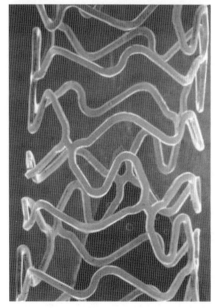

Figure 29.3: *Picture of stent by electron microscopy.*

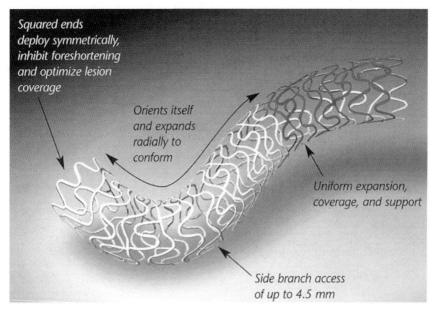

Squared ends deploy symmetrically, inhibit foreshortening and optimize lesion coverage

Orients itself and expands radially to conform

Uniform expansion, coverage, and support

Side branch access of up to 4.5 mm

Figure 29.4: Schematic drawing of the R Stent depicting its geometry and key features. Red indicates the dual helix backbone that is the main structure of the stent.

Coronary R stent technical specifications

Material composition:	316 L stainless steel
Degree of radiopacity (grade):	Moderate
Ferromagnetism:	Non-ferromagnetic (MRI safe)
MRI:	Safe
Metallic surface area	expanded: 12–18%
Stent design:	Dual helical slotted tube featuring three dimensional conformability and squared end-zones
Strut design:	Electropolished rectangular cross-section with rounded edges
Strut dimensions:	0.0039 inch (0.10 mm) 0.0050 inch (0.13 mm)
Strut thickness:	0.0050 inch (0.13 mm)
Profile(s): non-expanded (uncrimped): expanded: on the balloon:	Confidential Nominal pressure of 10 atm Crimped on balloon, 1.0 mm at 3.0 mm
Longitudinal flexibility:	Excellent
Percentage shortening (on delivery):	0%
Percentage shortening on expansion:	2.5–3.0 mm: < 1% 3.5–4.0 mm: < 3%
Expansion range:	2.5 mm–4.5 mm
Degree of recoil (shape memory):	< 3%
Radial force:	> 30 psi
Currently available diameters:	2.5, 2.75, 3.0, 3.5 and 4.0 mm
Currently available lengths mounted/implanted: unmounted:	9, 13, 18, & 23 mm @ 2.5 and 2.75 mm 9, 13, 18, 23, 28, & 33 mm @ 3.0 thru 4.0 mm
Currently available sizes:	9, 13, 18, 23 mm @ 2.5 and 2.75 mm 9, 13, 18, 23, 28, 33 mm @ 3.0 thru 4.0 mm
Recrossability of implanted stent:	Excellent
	Side branch access potentially to 4.5 mm, without deforming the stent
Other non-coronary types available:	In development

R Stent TALOS stent delivery system

Mechanism of deployment:	Balloon expandable
Design:	Rapid exchange
Guidewire compatibility:	0.014 inch (0.36 mm)
Minimum internal diameter of guiding catheter:	5 Fr
Crimped stent profile:	1.1 mm
Balloon characteristics:	High pressure, semi-compliant
Distance between edge of balloon and stent:	1 mm on each end of the stent
Rated burst pressure of balloon:	16 atm
Balloon compliance:	0.35 mm at 6 atm above nominal pressure
Protective sheath:	No
Available bare (unmounted):	Yes
Position of radiopaque markers:	(2) Proximal and distal to stent
Delivery system trackability:	Excellent

R Stent EVOLUTION stent delivery system

Mechanism of deployment:	Balloon expandable
Design:	Rapid exchange – hypotube
Guidewire compatibility:	0.014 inch (0.36 mm)
Minimum internal diameter of guiding catheter:	5 Fr
Crimped stent profile:	1.0 mm
Balloon characteristics:	High pressure, semi-compliant
Distance between edge of balloon and stent:	0.5 mm on each end of the stent
Rated burst pressure of balloon:	16 atm
Balloon compliance:	0.25 mm at 6 atm above nominal pressure
Protective sheath:	No
Available bare (unmounted):	Yes
Position of radiopaque markers:	(2) Proximal and distal to stent
Delivery system trackability:	Excellent

Indications for use

The R Stent is indicated for use in patients undergoing percutaneous revascularization of de novo and/or restenotic coronary artery lesions, associated with stable or unstable anginal symptoms.

As a result of its extremely high flexibility and radial strength, coupled with a low crossing profile the R Stent is especially useful for direct stenting without pre-dilatation and for both crossing through and stenting in tortuous coronary anatomy, as well as in ostial lesions. The large expandable cell size makes this product ideal for maintaining access to side branches and for stenting bifurcation lesions, where indicated.

Why I like my stent

I was initially intrigued by the 'DNA-like' double helical coil structure of the R stent, which actually renders it extremely longitudinally flexible, while at the same time boasting an unrivalled radial force. The potential 4.5 mm diameter side branch access through the struts is the icing on the cake. My initial experience in 1997 was with hand crimping the stent, which was challenging because of the need for patient and thorough unidirectional crimping, unlike other hand crimped stents. The retention of the crimped stent was extremely impressive and I have even performed direct stenting with it, in one instance during a live transmission in Uberlandia, Brazil, through a tortuous Circumflex. The Talos delivery system was somewhat bulkier than concurrent stents on the market, but the Evolution compares very favorably with currently available fourth and fifth generation systems. In my opinion, the R stent is a 'stent for all lesions', available from 2.5 to 4.0 mm in 9–33 mm, with plans for 4.5 mm and perhaps 5.0 mm diameter, to allow tailored stenting of left main lesions and lesions in larger coronaries and bypass grafts. In particular the R stent is very side branch friendly, with stenting across side branches rarely occluding or significantly impairing flow in the (non-significantly diseased side branch). Guidewire access to side branches after R stenting is usually easy, although occasionally bad fortune can leave a strut directly at the opening, requiring considerable catheter support and an ultra-low profile balloon to cross. However, having crossed the struts into the branch, a low-pressure inflation is usually enough to splay the struts apart and the outcome is reliably satisfactory. I have used the R stent frequently for 'culottes' type bifurcation stenting, often after first debulking with directional atherectomy, with extremely satisfying results (an example is shown here). The ease of crossing and re-crossing through the struts to the side branch is particularly appealing. I have also used the R stent for direct stenting of ostial side branch lesions, stenting across the ostium, into the main vessel (including stenting the ostial LAD into the left main, across the circumflex), then opening the struts in the direction of the main vessel and using kissing balloons to complete the job. I have rarely needed to stent the main vessel, because of dissection after kissing balloons. It was the availability of the R stent, with its double advantage of high radial force and excellent side branch access that provided me with the initial opportunity to apply this approach. In my opinion, this is an excellent, safe and rapid approach to treating important branch ostial lesions, which are notoriously difficult to stent accurately without either missing part of the ostium or protruding slightly into the main vessel, which can be especially troublesome in ostial LAD lesions, when future access to the circumflex needs to be secured.

I have also used the R stent for direct stenting of unprotected left main lesions and been able to expand the stent to 5 mm diameter (using IVUS guidance), showing impressive radial force. In heavily calcified lesions, the R stent has also shown impressive radial force in reaching full expansion in most cases.

At the time of writing, a cumulative total of more than 400 patients have been treated by R stents for a wide range of coronary lesions at the Thoraxcenter, Rotterdam. With no specific indications, systematic repeat angiography has not been performed, but clinical restenosis is < 10% overall, with data collection continuing. In the RESTOR registry, angiographic follow up of 125 patients treated for a single lesion will provide an initial figure for 6 month angiographic outcome and the DIRECTOR trial will provide data on the R stent for direct stenting. Developments are ongoing, specifically in the areas of stent coating, covered stents and peripheral R stents, all of which I eagerly await.

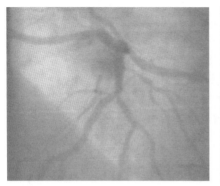

Figure 29.5: Pre-Intervention.

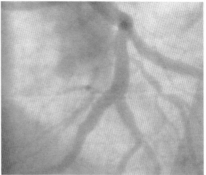

Figure 29.6: Post-R stent implantation.

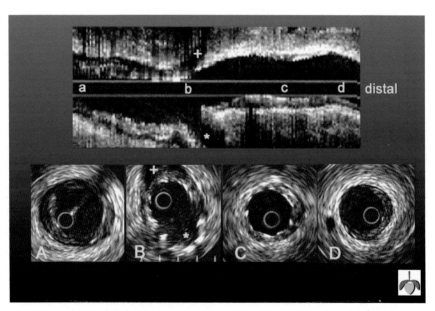

Figure 29.7: 6 Month – IVUS Follow-up. Image provided by Mr Jurgen Ligthart.

On-going or planned trials or registries

Center or study name and CRO	Number of patients	Principal	Follow-up investigator	Status or results
Royal Victoria Hospital Belfast, Northern Ireland 'Bifurcation Lesions'	28	M. Khan	1 year clinical follow-up complete *Single Center Registry*	Manuscript pending review
Ignatius Ziekenhuis Breda, The Netherlands 'Direct Stenting'	69	P. den Heijer	30 day clinical follow-up complete *Single Center Registry*	Manuscript pending review
RESTOR 'R Stent Efficacy and Safety Trial by Orbus' Cardialysis BV	121	P.W. Serruys	1 month clinical follow-up complete 6 month angiographic follow-up pending 9 month clinical follow-up pending *Multicenter Registry*	Results expected November 2001
DIRECTOR 'DIRECT stenting with the Orbus R stent' Cardialysis BV	120	B. Rensing	1 month clinical follow-up pending 6 month angiographic follow-up pending 9 month clinical follow-up pending *Multicenter Registry*	Results expected August 2002

30. THE RITHRON AND RITHRON-XR CORONARY STENTS

Biotronik GmbH, Berlin, Germany

Jacques Koolen, Hans Bonnier and Marcel Schaefer

Description	The Rithron (XR) coronary stent is a balloon-expandable tubular device cut from 316 L stainless steel. This flexible and conformable stent is coated with a thin hypothrombogenic coating of amorphous hydrogenated silicon carbide (a-SiC:H). For easier fluoroscopic visualization of the coronary stent there is an XR version with 2.0 mm ring radiopaque markers at the distal and proximal end of the stent. The Rithron (XR) is available as a bare stent (under the name Tenax and Tenax XR) and as a stent system, pre-mounted on a low-profile fast-exchange delivery system. The Rithron (XR) delivery systems are hypotube based and 5 Fr guiding catheter compatible.

History	• Early 1997 first human implantations • Spring 1997 single centre registry • Spring 1999 introduction of Tenax XR with superior fluoroscopic visibility • September 1999 introduction of Tenax XR[Trinity], a multi-balloon indirect primary stenting system • September 2000 introduction of Teneo, a new hypotube based stent delivery system • May 2001 introduction of Rithron, a new improved hypotube-based stent delivery system

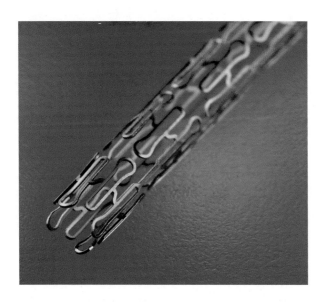

Figure 30.1:
Rithron 316L tubular slotted design coated with a-SiC:H. The geometry shows connecting articulations in combination with 'keyholes' in opposite orientations to increase flexibility/ conformability and the functionality of the stent.

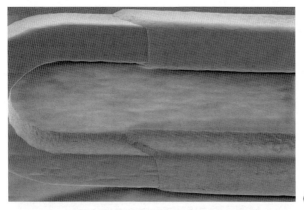

(a)

Figure 30.2:
Transition from the 2 mm gold-plated end-segment to the pure 316 L surface on a Rithron stent. Both surfaces are homogeneously coated with a-SiC:H.
(a) unexpanded and
(b) expanded.

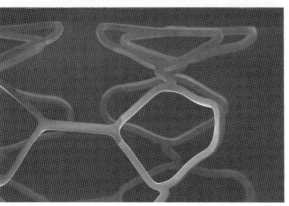

(b)

Rithron/Rithron-XR stent specifications

Material composition:	316 L stainless steel coated with hypothrombogenic a-SiC:H
Stent design:	Tubular slotted
Strut thickness:	0.0031 inch/0.08 mm/80 μm
Thickness of coating:	~0.08 μm
Radiopacity mid-section:	Low to moderate
Radiopacity end-sections:	Low to moderate (Rithron), high (Rithron-XR)
Metallic surface area:	14%
Shortening:	3%
Flexibility of crimped stent:	Very high
Conformability:	Highly conformable
Mechanical recoil:	≤ 5%
Ferromagnetism/MRI:	Non ferromagnetic, MRI safe
Available lengths:	10, 15, 20, 25, 30 mm
Expansion range:	2.5–4.5 mm

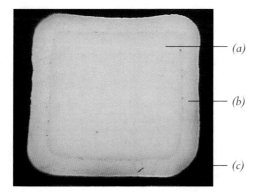

(a)

(b)

(c)

Figure 30.3: Gold plating of the end-segments of the Rithron-XR stent. (a) 80 μm 316L stainless steel; (b) 7 μm gold plating; (c) 0.08 μm a-SiC:H layer.

Rithron/Rithron-XR stent delivery system

Catheter type:	Fast exchange
Proximal shaft:	2.1 Fr, Hypotube, BIOCoating
Distal shaft:	2.5 Fr/2.7 Fr HDPE, Hydro X-plus coating
Longitudinal flexibility:	High
Minimal ID of GC:	0.055 inch (1.40 mm)
Mechanism of expansion:	PropWrap
Balloon material:	TELL (semicompliant)
Position of radiopaque balloon markers:	Proximal and distal to stent
Stent fixation:	New stent/balloon fixation
Recommended expansion pressure:	8–10 atm
Nominal pressure:	6 atm
Rated burst pressure:	12–16 atm
Balloon lengths:	12, 17, 22, 27 and 32 mm
Diameters available:	2.5–4.0 mm
Delivery profile:	2.5 mm–0.042 inch (1.07 mm) 3.0 mm–0.044 inch (1.12 mm) 3.5 mm–0.044 inch (1.12 mm) 4.0 mm–0.044 inch (1.12 mm)

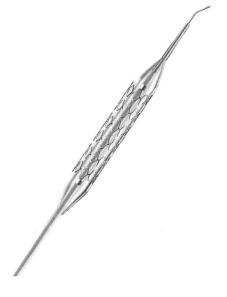

Figure 30.4: *The inflated Rithron-XR stent system.*

Rithron/Rithron-XR coronary stent system

The Rithron delivery system is made from a 2.1 Fr proximal hypotube, coated with BIOCoating. The new designed shaft has a shorter transition length for improved pushability and the distal shaft is coated with hydrophilic Hydro X-Plus coating. In addition the Rithron features a new crimping method which makes it extremely safe for direct stenting.

Indications for use

The Rithron coronary stent can be used in both native coronary arteries or bypass grafts. The low crossing profile of Rithron combined with reliable stent fixation, high stent retention force, hypothrombogenic a-SiC:H surface coating and full lesion assimilation provide for high clinical success rates in direct or indirect stenting applications (in suitable lesions). Good visualization of the proximal and distal stent ends enables precise placement as required for ostial and bifurcation lesions. The geometry of the tubular slotted design of the Rithron stent enable moderate to good side branch access. Due to the range of stent lengths available (10–30 mm) a wide range of lesions can be treated.

Why I like my stent

- The high flexibility and low profile of the design provides Rithron with balloon-like handling characteristics enabling easy and rapid delivery in tortuous vessels
- The hypothrombogenic a-SiC:H coating reduces the risk of thrombotic stent occlusion and sub-acute thrombotic events
- Optimal stent to vessel ratio is possible due to the broad range of different lengths and diameter sizes
- If desired, manual crimping is quick and easy to perform
- Rithron can be introduced through guiding catheters with an ID of 0.055 inch
- Positioning is facilitated by two radiopaque ring markers at both ends of the stent (Rithron XR)
- The Rithron stent has been associated with attractively low target vessel revascularization rates in clinical practice in unselected patient groups
- With the new delivery system the handling of Rithron is safe and successful in almost any anatomy.

Tips and tricks for delivery

The bare stent version is quick and easily mounted onto standard PTCA balloons by hand with no special tool required. The pre-mounted Rithron has the stent firmly positioned on the balloon by the stent seating platform. The PropWrap expansion of the delivery balloons optimizes the symmetrical radial expansion of the stent during the deployment phase. Rithron can be easily delivered through a 5 Fr guiding catheter with an inner lumen ≥ 0.055 inch.

Ongoing and planned trials

- A multicenter study to evaluate the safety and efficacy of the Rithron-XR is currently ongoing in the USA.

Completed trials

- TRUST study with 485 patients in an international multi-centre randomized trial with IVUS and QCA follow-up to compare Tenax XR with silicon carbide coating to standard non-coated 316 L stainless steel stents in acute coronary syndromes. Preliminary results show significant clinical benefit for high risk patients. Final results presented at ESC 2001.
- SVS small vessel multi-centre European study commenced summer 1998 with 500 patients randomized to stent implantation using Tenax XR or balloon angioplasty in small vessels (≤ 3.0 mm). World's largest study on small calibre vessels. Recruitment completed, and expected to be published in 2001. The results clearly demonstrate the advantage of the silicon carbide coating as compared to stainless steel stents.
- TENISS trial to investigate the hypothesis that the semiconducting properties of a-SiC:H coating reduces acute and sub-acute stent thrombosis in everyday clinical practice compared to uncoated stainless steel stents. Published ESC 2000.
- The BET Trial (Benefit Evaluation of direct Coronary Stenting), a randomized French multicentre trial, shows feasibility of direct stenting with the Tenax coronary stent and a reduction of procedural cost and length (*Am J Cardiol* 2001; **87**: 693–698).

Review of the literature

Despite the use of IVUS, high pressure inflation and improved antiplatelet protocols, (sub)acute stent thrombosis remains a potentially lethal complication of stent implantation. To decrease the risk of stent thrombosis and other unfavourable events, the haemocompatibility of a stent is determined by its surface properties. Smooth surfaces are necessary to avoid the activation of the clotting cascade via trapped blood components. However, different materials with the same surface roughness affect the clotting system differently.[1] Thrombogenesis on an artificial surface is induced by an electron transfer from fibrinopeptide to the solid stainless steel surface.[2] If an electron tunnels from a blood clotting protein—especially fibrinogen—to an alloplastic material, the protein changes its tertiary structure, which results in clotting.[3] To prevent fibrin deposition and thrombus formation on the stent surface, the electronic transfer current from fibrinogen to stent surface must be minimized. Hydrogen rich amorphous silicon carbide (a-SiC:H) is a semiconductor with favourable properties. In vitro testing showed that a-SiC:H did not cause a cytotoxic reaction or haemolysis. The Ames test demonstrated that the number of mutagenic cells caused by a-SiC:H is the same as that caused by saline, so no mutagenic affect can be attributed to a-SiC:H. Scanning electron microscopy showed complete coverage of the stent surface with endothelial cells.[4] Comparison of an uncoated stent and an a-SiC:H coated stent explanted 90 minutes after implantation in a pig carotid artery showed reduced blood component aggregation on an a-SiC:H coated stent.[5] First clinical experience with the Tenax stent demonstrated high functionality, excellent handling characteristics and promising initial clinical results.[6] These were confirmed in the TRUST study and a recent French multicentre registry where 241 unselected patients were treated with the Tenax stent. Procedural success (97.4%) and clinical success (95.4%) were high. Only 7.2% of patients needed target lesion revascularization after 12 months follow-up.[7]

References

1. Bolz A, Amon M, Ozbek C *et al*. Optimization of hemocompatibility and functionality by a hybrid design of cardiovascular stents. *Prog in Biomed Res* 1996:8–12.

2. Baurschmidt P, Schaldach M. The electrochemical aspects of the thrombogenicity of a material. *J Bioeng* 1977;1:261–78.

3. Bolz A. Physikalische Mechanismen der Festkörper-Protein-Wechselwirkung un der Phasen-grenze a-SiC:H-Fibrinogen. PhD thesis at the University of Erlangen, Germany 1991.

4. Bolz A, Amon M, Ozbek C *et al*. Coating of cardiovascular stents with a semiconductor to improve their hemocompatibility. *Tex Heart Inst J* 1996;23:162–6.

5. Amin M, Bolz A, Heublein B *et al*. Coating of cardiovascular stents with amorphous silicon carbide to reduce thrombogenicity. *Proceedings of the 16th Annual Conference of the IEEE Engineering in Medicine and Biology Society*, 1994; 838.

6. Koolen J, Hanekamp C, Bonnier H. A highly flexible slotted tube stent design coated with a-SiC:H first clinical experience. *Prog in Biomed Res* 1998;2.

7. Carrie D, Khalife K, Hamon M et al. Initial and follow-up results of the Tenax coronary stent. *J Interv Cardiol* 2001;14:1–5.

31. THE SEAQUEST™ STENT

CathNet-Science SA, Paris, France

Philippe Rossi

Description	The Seaquest™ stent is a third generation stent. It is the successor to the Seaquence™ stent and combines the radial resistance of a tubular stent with the flexibility and vessel wall comformability of a modular or coil stent. CathNet-Science's development goal was to combine in the same design, the following technical parameters:

- Optimal vessel scaffolding
- Optimal stent flexibility and conformability to the vessel wall
- Optimal radial resistance

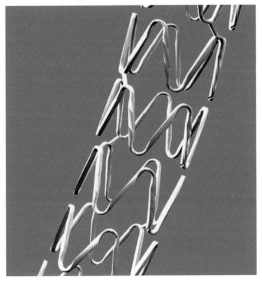

Figure 31.1: *Expanded Seaquest™ stent.*

The Seaquest™ stent is a balloon expandable stainless steel, tubular stent. It is designed as a series of rings, each with repeating 'S' shape. Each ring is connected to its neighbour by a single oblique and asymmetrically placed bridge. As a result, the expansion of this stent design shows zigzag corrugations in parallel. The smaller stents (2.5 and 3.0 mm) are designed with five cells and the larger diameters (3.5 and 4.0 mm) are designed with six cells. This differentiated design ensures comparable cell distribution and metal surface area in vessels of different sizes.

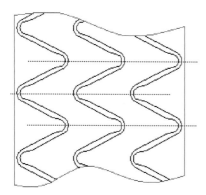

Figure 31.2: *Seaquest™ expansion design.*

These zigzag corrugations and links between segments introduced in an asymmetric rotating configuration provide an optimal longitudinal flexibility. This permits easy access to very distal lesions even in tortuous anatomy. Furthermore, the large cell size allows side branch patency.

Delivery system

The Seaquest™ stent is mounted on a new PTCA balloon catheter range: Searider Sensitive®. This is a balloon with improved trackability, pushability and crossability qualities. The balloon is made of a semi-compliant material which allows controlled sizing and post-dilatation. The balloon has a high rated burst pressure (RBP 16 atm) which allows high pressure stent implantation or post-dilatation. The 3-fold balloon configuration ensures a symmetric stent expansion. The 3-fold shape memory allows for excellent rewrapping and ensures a low balloon profile in case recrossing and redilatation are necessary.

Seaquest™ stent specifications

Diameters:	2.5, 3.0, 3.5, 4.0 mm
Stent lengths:	8, 12, 18, 28, 38 mm
Balloon lengths:	12, 15, 20, 30, 40 mm
Design:	Slotted tube
Material:	Stainless steel 316 L
Sterilization method:	Ethylene oxide
Ferromagnetism:	Non-ferromagnetic
% Metal/artery:	From 12 to 17%
Strut thickness:	0.13 mm/0.005 inch
Foreshortening (average):	<3%
Recoil:	<4%
Radial force:	Good
Mechanism of deployment:	Balloon
Mounted profiles:	
2.5 mm	1.00 mm/0.039 inch
3.0 mm	1.05 mm/0.041 inch
3.5 mm	1.21 mm/0.048 inch
4.0 mm	1.27 mm/0.050 inch
Radiopacity:	Good
Longitudinal flexibility:	Excellent

Searider Sensitive® balloon specifications

Type:	Rapid exchange
Total length:	140 cm
Proximal shaft diameter:	1.8 Fr
Medial shaft diameter:	2.6 Fr
Distal part diameter:	2.8 Fr
Crossing profile:	0.018 inch
Tip length:	3.5 mm
Internal tube inner lumen:	0.017 inch
Coating:	Hydrophilic coating
Radiopaque markers:	Two: proximal and distal to the stent
Balloon resistance:	
Nominal size	6 atm
Rated Burst Pressure	16 atm
Average Burst Pressure	22 atm

Seaquest™ clinical case and comments

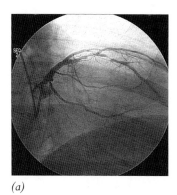

(a)

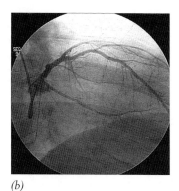

(b)

Figure 31.3(a): *Diffuse critical stenosis (>20 mm long) of the mid-LAD treated via the radial approach. Note the small diagonal branch originating from the middle of the lesion.*

Figure 31.3(b): *Post-stenting result with a Seaquest™ 3.0/38 mm long. Note the conformability of the stent to the curvature of the LAD and the good patency of the side branch.*

Indications for use

Recognized use of intracoronary stents currently includes, but is not limited to, the treatment of de novo or restenotic lesions in native coronary arteries and de novo lesions in saphenous vein grafts. The Seaquest™ is available for intracoronary implantation vessel diameters of 2.5 to 4.0 mm.

Why I like this stent

The Seaquest™ metallic coronary stent is a third generation stent which combines the potential advantages of radial strength, good flexibility and conformability to the vessel wall. It is premounted on a very low profile semi-compliant latest generation PTCA balloon catheter: the Searider Sensitive®. This has permitted a significant improvement in the crossing profile of the stent compared to the former CathNet-Science stent, the Seaquence™. The Seaquest™ is available in a usual range of diameters (from 2.5 to 4 mm) and various lengths from short (8 mm) to very long (38 mm) stents including intermediate lengths of 12, 18 and 28 mm. Since its launch at the end of October 2000, we have implanted more than 100 Seaquest™ stents. This preliminary experience with the routine use of the stent showed several major advantages:

- The very low profile of the Seaquest™/Searider® system confers high crossing power even in complex and tortuous anatomy. This is particularly useful for direct stenting, which constitutes 40–50% of our cases.
- The excellent trackability and pushability of the Seaquest™ stent allows us to reach distal lesions in complex cases and in calcified vessels.
- Excellent flexibility and conformability to the vessel wall, especially when stenting in coronary curves.
- Stent design permits excellent side-branch access, very useful for bifurcation lesions or stenting by a collateral. The stent can be recrossed.

Ongoing studies

Name	Number of patients	Endpoints	Type	Status	Results
European Clinical Observation Seaquence™ conducted by Pr Hamon CHU Caen, France	161 • Multicenter • Europe	• Primary endpoint MACE and TLR at 1 month and 9 month follow-up • Secondary endpoint: procedural success rate	• Registry • Clinical Follow up	Complete 1 and 9 month data available	Publication: on-going
Israeli Seaquence™ Registry conducted by the Israeli Working Group for Interventional Cardiology	107 • Multicenter • Israel	• MACE at 1 month and 6 months	• Registry • Clinical Follow up	Complete 6 month follow up data available	MACE at 1 month: Rehospitalization: 1% for a CABG MACE at 6 months: Death: 2% Rehospitalization: 15% Recatheterization: 14% Open artery: 3% Unsuccessful: 2%
DISCUSS Study Austria (Direct Stenting In Coronaries Using the Seaquence™ Stent)	300 (2 groups) • Multicenter • Austria	• Primary endpoint: safety and procedural success rate • Secondary endpoint: investigate the short- and long-term results of the primary stenting, the prevalence of stent restenosis and the occurrence of major cardiac events	• Randomized study • Angiographic control	On-going	
Direct Coronary Stenting without predilatation using the Seaquence™ Stent Italy – Turin	115 • Multicenter • Italy	• Primary endpoint: safety and procedural success rate • Secondary endpoint: MACE at 3 months and 6 months	• Registry • Clinical follow-up at 3 months and 6 months • Treadmill stress test at 6 months	Complete Data available	• Overall success of direct implantation of the Seaquence stent: 92% • 1 month follow-up: overall success rate: 99% • Follow-up at 20 weeks: TVR 9% (12 patients)

Name	Number of patients	Endpoints	Type	Status	Results
European Clinical Observation Seaquest™ Stent conducted by the Centre Hospitalier Privé Clairval in Marseille – Dr Rossi	215 • Multicenter • Europe	• Primary endpoint: MACE and TLR at 1 month and 6 months follow-up • Secondary endpoint: procedural success rate	• Registry • Clinical follow-up	Complete • Data at 1 month available • Follow-up at 6 months on-going	• 245 stents were successfully implanted • During hospital stay, MACE were seen in 6 patients MI in 6 patients (2.8%) Repeat PTCA in 1 patient (0.5%) for a sub-acute stent thrombosis No death and no coronary bypass Bleeding or vascular complication were seen in 2 patients (0.9%) • MACE at 1 month: 1 coronary bypass for 1 patient for recurrent ischemia TLR: 0.47% • 6 month follow-up: on-going

32. THE SPIRAL FORCE STENT

Bolton Medical Inc. Fair Lawn, NJ, USA

Norman T Kanesaka and Tomás Berrazueta

Definition	The Spiral Force coronary stent is a tubular stent, which is cut from 316 L stainless steel and electro-polished. It features a unique spiral strut design in which all of the struts are connected with inverted C-joints. This spiral design provides unsurpassed flexibility, while the connection of all struts ensures uniform expansion and a high radial force. The stent offers outstanding radial force and minimum recoil, because the scaffolding design connects all struts together for uniform distribution of support.

History	Introduced in 1999 and distributed worldwide since then. The Spiral Force's unique spiral design provides excellent flexibility.

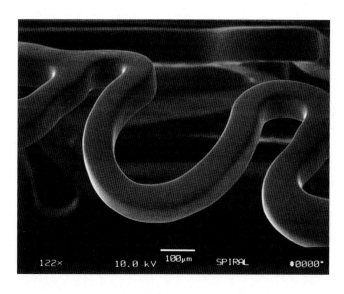

Figure 32.1:
Electron micrograph of Spiral Force Stent.

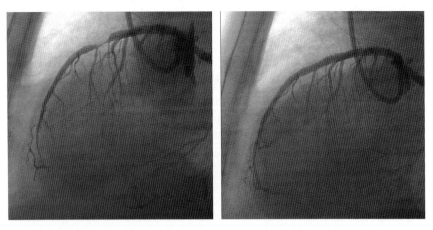

Figure 32.2: *Spiral Force Stent, pre- and post-LAD implantation.*

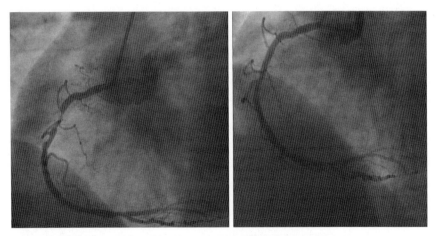

Figure 32.3: *Spiral Force Stent, pre- and post-RCA implantation.*

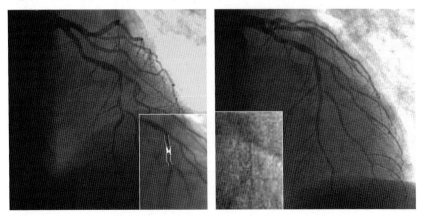

Figure 32.4: *Spiral Force Stent, pre- and post-LAD implantation.*

268

Spiral Force stent technical specifications

Material composition:	316 L stainless steel
Degree of radiopacity (grade):	Moderate
Ferromagnetism:	Non-Ferromagnetic
MRI:	MRI Safe
Stent design:	Spiral cut with C-joints
Strut design:	Straight struts
Strut dimensions:	0.005 inch × 0.026 inch to 0.005 inch × 0.035 inch
Strut angles:	40°–45° 4 mm internal diameter
Strut thickness:	0.003 inch
Wire thickness:	Not applicable
Mesh angle:	Not applicable
Mesh braid angle:	Not applicable
Profile(s): non-expanded (uncrimped):	0.067 inch
expanded:	2.7 to 4.2 mm
on the balloons:	0.039 inch to 0.042 inch
Longitudinal flexibility:	Excellent
Percentage shortening on expansion:	3.8–8.2% depending an expansion
Expansion range:	2.5 mm to 4.25 mm
Degree of recoil (shape memory):	1.2%
Radial force:	Very high
Currently available diameters:	2.5, 3.0, 3.5, 4.0 mm
Currently available lengths mounted/unmounted:	9, 13, 17, 21 and 27
Other non-coronary types available:	Femoral, iliac, renal in late 2001

Delivery system

The rapid exchange Runner is the latest generation stent delivery balloon catheter. The Zylite balloon material (semi-compliant) gives: controlled compliance, increased flexibility, optimal refolding and high pressure seating.

The Runner balloon is also designed to be used for standard PTCA procedures, such as routine pre-dilatation angioplasty and post-stent deployment. It is available in all lengths and diameters.

Tips and tricks for delivery

This is a really simple stent to use due to the adequate radiopacity and flexibility. Due to the low compliance of the balloon and the easy stent expansion at mid-pressures, it is recommended to slightly oversize the stent. It is unusual to observe distal dissections. All sizes of the Spiral Force stent can be easily delivered through all commercially available 6 Fr guiding catheters and through a Medtronic Zuma 5 Fr guiding catheter.

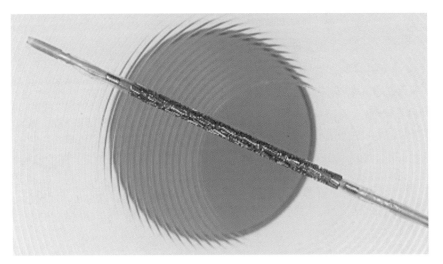

Figure 32.5: Spiral Force premounted on the Runner delivery system.

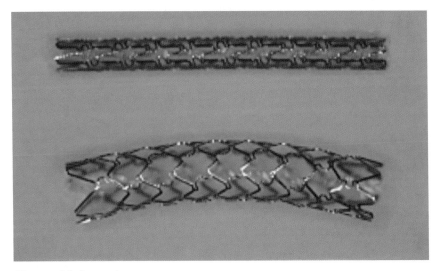

Figure 32.6: Spiral Force stent.

Indications for use

The Spiral Force (SF)™ balloon-expandable stent is indicated for use in de novo native coronary artery lesions with a reference vessel diameter in the range of 2.5–4 mm and a length up to 25 mm. In this population, stenting produces a larger luminal diameter, maintains arterial patency, and reduces the incidence of restenosis at six months as compared with balloon angioplasty. One year and longer follow-up is not well characterized.

Why I like my stent

There are many specifications for stents, but three major factors – flexibility, radial force and recoil – play the major roles in short and long term performance of the stent. Flexibility can be obtained either by design configuration or skipping connections. Higher radial force can be achieved from using a thicker material or connecting all struts. Reduced recoil rate is a design and material issue. The Spiral Force stent successfully comprises all three factors.

The Spiral Force achieves all three goals with superior engineering without compromising other factors nor resorting to the easier solutions.

Studies in which stent is involved

1) JAPAN:
   Japanese Spiral Force Study – 100 Patients (Finished)
2) SPAIN + PORTUGAL:
   RESET (Spiral Force Spanish Registry) – 428 Patients (Finished)
3) BELGIUM:
   SPIFO (Spiral Force Patency, Belgium Study) – 75 Patients (Running)
4) FRANCE:
   Spiral Force French Registry – 125 Patients (Running)

33. THE TSUNAMI CORONARY STENT SYSTEM

Terumo Corporation, Japan

Masakiyo Nobuyoshi

Description	• Balloon expandable
	• Stainless steel slotted tube stent
	• Double-linked diamond cell structure

Important features of Tsunami

- **Superb deliverability**
  Hydrophilic M coat™ is applied onto the tip and distal shaft of the delivery balloon catheter, decreasing friction when moistened. In addition to the M coat™, the benefits of the ultra-low profile (0.038 inch for 3.0 mm system), the unique double-link connection, the smooth stent surface, and the Tri-fold balloon combine to ensure superb stent delivery, trackability and crossability.
- **Exceptional conformability**
  Terumo's double-link structure — diamond-shaped cells joined by two connectors — results in unequalled stent flexibility. This pliable stent gives exceptional conformability to natural tortuosity of coronary vessels once deployed.
- **Powerful and stable radial force**
  Radial strength and vessel coverage on bends are assured by the stainless steel laser-cut tube design and the double-link cell pattern. When placed in the lesion, the stent firmly retains its shape and position.
- **Minimum injury and maximum security**
  Tsunami's minimal balloon overhang (< 1 mm) lessens injury during dilatation. In addition, the stent edge design reduces flaring risk providing more secure procedure.

Tsunami technical specifications

Material composition:	316 L stainless steel
Degree of radiopacity:	Moderate
Ferromagnetism:	Moderate
MRI:	Safe
Metallic surface area expanded:	< 18%
Stent design:	Several radial diamonds joined by double connector
Strut design:	Square
Strut thickness:	0.08 mm
Non-expanded profile:	0.95 mm (0.038 inch) for the 3.0 mm stent system
Longitudinal flexibility:	Excellent
Percentage shortening:	< 5%
Degree of recoil:	< 5%
Current available sizes:	2.5/15, 2.5/20, 2.5/30
	3.0/10, 3.0/15, 3.0/20, 3.0/30
	3.5/10, 3.5/15, 3.5/20, 3.5/30
	4.0/10, 4.0/15, 4.0/20
Other non-coronary types available:	None

Tsunami stent delivery system

Mechanism of deployment:	Balloon expandable
Minimal internal diameter of guiding catheter:	0.056 inch, 5 Fr
Pre-mounted on delivery catheter	Yes
Protective sheath/cover:	No
Position of radiopaque markers:	Distal and proximal to stent
Recommended deployment pressure:	Nominal at 10 atm (9 atm for 4.0 mm)
Further balloon expansion recommended	Discretionary
Supply in bare	No
Recrossability of deployed stent	Good
Sizing diameter	Equal to artery or over-sizing up to 10%

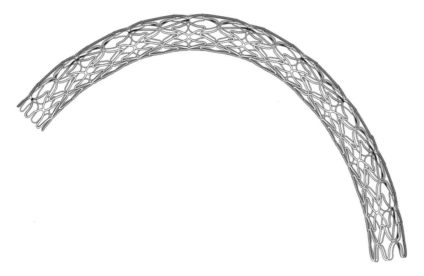

Figure 33.1: Tsunami — conformability.

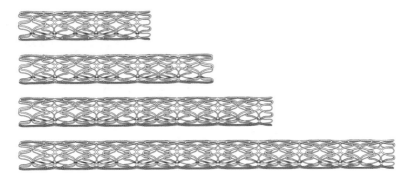

Figure 33.2: Tsunami product range (10, 15, 20 and 30 mm lengths).

275

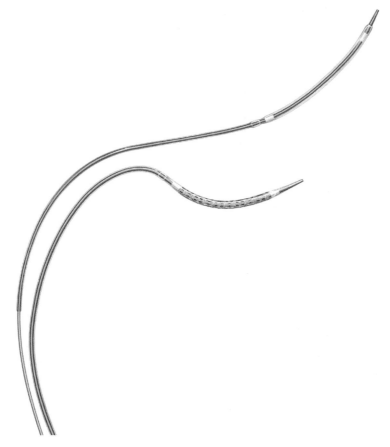

Figure 33.3: *Tsunami delivery system.*

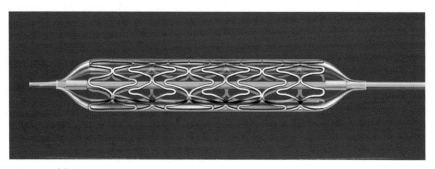

Figure 33.4: *Expanded Tsunami stent system.*

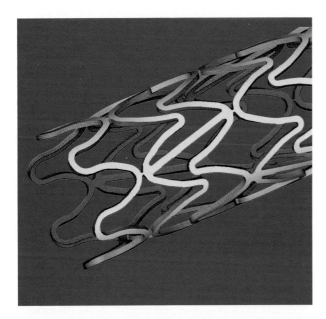

Figure 33.5:
Expanded Tsunami stent.

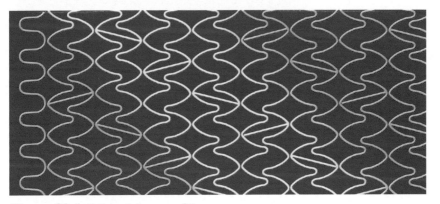

Figure 33.6: *Technical drawing of Tsunami.*

Indications for use

- Useful in distal and tortuous vessel
- Long lesions
- Acute closure or bail out situations
- Smaller vessels
- Acute myocardial infarction
- De-novo lesions
- Lesions in bends
- Vein graft stenosis
- Sub-optimal PTCA result
- Moderate calcified lesions

Why I like my stent

- Superior deliverability assured by very low profile (one of the lowest), M coat (Terumo's hydrophilic polymer on tip and shaft), and flexible system (unique double-link connection).
- Good conformability and high radial force for long-term outcome provided by double-linked diamond cells tubular structure.
- Minimum vessel injury realized by minimal balloon overhang.

Ongoing planned trials

- Japan trial, Dr Masakiyo Nobuyoshi, Kokura Memorial Hospital, Japan
- TESTER, Professor Serruys, Thoraxcenter, Rotterdam, The Netherlands

Review of the current published literature

- Nobuyoshi M, Yokoi H, Mitsudo K, Kadota K, Saito S, Hosokawa J. Early and late outcomes of Coronary Stent System (TRE-963). *J Clin Exp Med* 1998;**75**:209–221.
- Yokoi H, Nakagawa Y, Tamura T, Hamasaki N, Kimura T, Nosaka H, Nobuyoshi M. Preliminary experiences with the Terumo coronary stent [abstract]. *J Am Coll Cardiol* 1998;**31**(suppl):413A.

34. THE ZEBRA STENT

Bolton Medical Inc, Fair Lawn, NJ, USA

Norman T Kanesaka and Tomás Berrazueta

Definition	The Zebra coronary stent is a tubular stent, which is laser cut from 316 L stainless steel and electro-polished. It has bigger cells on both ends to give a 'variable metal coverage'. The central part features a spiral strut design in which all of the stents are connected with inverted C joints.

History	The Zebra was developed in mid-2000 to incorporate all the superior features of Bolton Medical's Spiral Force stent – flexibility, high radial force and minimum recoil – with reduced metal coverage on the stent ends for better transitions to the non-stented areas.

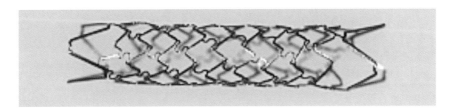

Figure 34.1: *Expanded Zebra stent.*

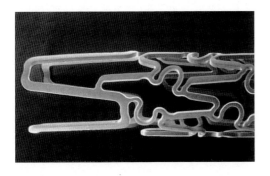

Figure 34.2: *Scanning electron micrograph of the Zebra stent.*

Zebra stent technical specifications

Material composition:	316 L stainless steel
Degree of radiopacity (grade):	Moderate
Ferromagnetism:	Non-ferromagnetic
MRI:	MRI safe
Metallic surface area expanded:	Approximately 13% at 3.5 mm
Stent design:	Spiral cut with C-joints
Strut design:	Straight struts
Strut dimensions:	0.005 inch × 0.026 inch to 0.007 inch × 0.080 inch
Strut angles:	40° to 55° @ 4 mm internal diameter
Strut thickness:	0.003 inch
Wire thickness:	Not Applicable
Mesh angle:	Not applicable
Mesh braid angle:	Not applicable
Profile(s): non-expanded (uncrimped): expanded: on the balloons:	0.067 inch 2.7 mm to 4.2 mm 0.039 inch to 0.042 inch
Longitudinal flexibility:	Excellent
Percentage shortening on expansion:	2.5–10.8% depending on expansion
Expansion range:	2.5 mm to 4.25 mm
Degree of recoil (shape memory):	1.2%
Radial force:	Very high
Currently available diameters:	2.5, 3.0, 3.5, 4.0 mm
Currently available lengths mounted/implanted: unmounted:	See tables 14 mm, 19 mm

Device for delivery

The rapid exchange Runner is the latest generation stent delivery balloon catheter. The Zylite balloon material (semi-compliant) gives: controlled compliance, increased flexibility, optimal refolding and high pressure seating.

The Runner balloon is also designed to be used for standard PTCA procedures, such as routine pre-dilatation angioplasty and post-stent deployment. It is available in all lengths and diameters.

Indications for use

See Spiral Force chapter.

Why I like my stent

The Zebra inherits all of the superior, fundamental design patterns of Bolton Medical's Spiral Force in the center of the stent, but the end cells are enlarged for reduced metal coverage. This is a very unique design.

Studies in which stent is involved

1) ZEBRA BELGIUM STUDY
   7 centres
   150 patients
   Registry
   Will start on June 2001

2) ZEBRA SPAIN STUDY
   5 centres
   200 patients
   Registry
   Will start on June 2001

DRUG-ELUTING STENTS

35. The Background, Rationale for and Current Status of the ELUTES (EvaLUation of paclitaxel Eluting Stent) Trial

Anthony H Gershlick and Ivan de Scheerder

Background

The development of significant atheromatous plaque narrowing in coronary arteries has a major impact on population morbidity and mortality and thus on health resources. While, ideally, the aim should be the prevention of the plaque formation in the first place, until a cost effective programme of early detection and prevention is available, treatment of the consequences of atheromatous plaque development will continue to play a major role in limiting patient symptoms and altering the natural history of the disease.

Management of coronary atheromatous narrowing has shifted from surgical to percutaneous intervention. Coronary angioplasty and stenting has become a commonplace treatment for patients with symptomatic coronary disease. Procedure rates vary from 450/million population to 3000/million. Worldwide these add up to nearly 1.5 million procedures per annum. While balloon angioplasty and stenting have in general a favourable outcome (>90%) primary success rate, the medium and longer term outcome may be influenced by the response of the vessel wall to injury.

The sequence of pathological events following coronary intervention

The sequence of changes following damage to the vessel wall has been well documented. These changes culminate in recurrence or restenosis and the need, because of luminal renarrowing, for further intervention. Balloon angioplasty causes deep damage to the vessel wall.[1–2] Endothelial denudation, intimal disruption and medial layer damage occur. Adventitial layer damage is thought to play an important role in the changes that are subsequently seen in the intimal layer. Plaque compression and stretch of non-atheromatous wall are the likely immediate effective mechanisms for the apparent benefit seen following balloon inflation. The subsequent repair process is complex with inflammatory and thrombotic pathways being activated. Platelets become adherent to the damaged vessel wall within seconds due to loss of protective endothelium and exposure of platelet to activating subendothelial collagen and basement membrane. Activation of platelets causes expression of the glycoprotein IIb/IIIa receptor. Coagulation pathways result in the formation of fibrinogen which, through the glycoprotein IIb/IIIa receptor, cross-links platelets. Thrombin, which is also formed, is a powerful stimulant of platelet activation and stimulus to medial cell proliferation. Formed thrombus is incorporated into the disrupted lesion, contributing to the restenotic process.[3] Activated platelets release growth factors that alter the medial smooth muscle cell (SMC) behaviour. White cell adhesion, adherent thrombin and growth factors from the smooth muscle cells themselves all contribute to the cellular phenotypic changes seen. There is early expression of nucleotides that initiate the change from G0 (quiescent) phase to G1 (proliferative phase). Factors such as TGF-β, IGF[4] and the angiotensin receptor on smooth muscle cells all contribute to the migratory and proliferative process. Animal data suggests a pivotal role for platelet-derived growth factor BB.[5] Migration through the disrupted internal elastic lamina into the thin intima is an important prelude to proliferation and metalloproteinases play an important role in lesion development at this time.[6]

Cellular changes and other factors leading to restenosis

An important factor in initiation and promotion of the restenotic response is de-endothelialization. Conversely, re-endothelialization can result in EDRF-induced SMC inhibition and cessation of exposure of the SMC to PDGF-BB and platelets. Re-endothelialization can take up to 2 weeks to complete, however, by which time the cellular processes leading to restenosis will have been initiated. The restenotic process is usually complete within 4–6 months. There is evidence, albeit indirect, that inhibition of these early processes can lead to longer term inhibition of the cellular changes.[7] It is also clear that there are many targets if one wished to inhibit the early phases of the restenotic process. Knowledge of such targets may be important when deciding on which agent to load onto a stent.

Tissue changes account for about 40–50% of the restenotic process following balloon angioplasty alone. It has been shown that while these tissue changes are important other factors also play a critical role in recurrence. Mintz[8] and others using intravascular ultrasound have described the process of negative remodelling whereby the development of the restenotic lesion itself contributes to contraction of the artery. The changes in external elastic membrane dimensions may be related to the effects of the balloon on wall structure, particularly following deep injury when the adventitia layer is damaged.

Altering the factors that lead to restenosis

Balloon angioplasty

Deploying stents with high radial strength has largely dealt with the problem of recoil[9] and negative remodelling. Clinical trials have shown that stenting reduces the incidence of restenosis,[10,11] with rates 10–15% lower following stenting compared to angioplasty. However, use of stents clearly has not abolished restenosis. Tissue growth still occurs within the stent. The rate of in-stent restenosis is influenced by a number of factors, predominantly the extent of the stimulus (multiple stents and stenting after significant intervention, such as opening chronic total occlusions), the size of the vessel (small arteries can accommodate the tissue responses less) and conditions where excess smooth muscle cell response occurs (diabetics). In these patients the in-stent restenosis rate is not 10–15% but nearer 30%. The factors can be additive.[12–18] A diabetic patient with a stent deployed in a coronary artery of small calibre might expect an in-stent restenosis rate of up to 50%.[19] Treatment of in-stent restenosis is difficult and re-restenosis for diffuse disease treated with balloon angioplasty may be up to 80%.[20] Rates of re-restenosis over 60% are commonly published.

Dealing with in-stent restenosis

Re-restenosis rates after repeat ballooning may be particularly high if the restenotic tissue is diffusely distributed throughout the stent. Reballooning diffuse in-stent restenosis has little longer term value. Tissue debulking treatments such as atherectomy were proposed, but benefit has not been demonstrated in the recently published ARTIST trial. Another therapeutic strategy is to deliver either β or γ radiation therapy to the stented artery and in a number of important trials this has been shown to reduce intimal tissue responses. Future proposals may include prophylactical treatment of those patients known to have a high risk of in-stent restenosis (diabetics, small vessels), but current practice is to wait until restenosis and administer the brachytherapy following reballooning. Problems with the use of brachytherapy include the delayed re-endothelialization that occurs due to cellular radiosensitivity, which in turn can increase the risk of stent thrombosis.[21] Most importantly, vascular brachytherapy is secondary treatment whereas what is needed is primary prevention of the in-stent restenotic process.

Inhibition of the restenotic process with drugs

More than 30 clinical trials of systemic agents were tested in the setting of balloon angioplasty restenosis. In general the results were disappointing. This may be explained by a number of factors; some of the studies were poorly designed, some were underpowered and sometimes the wrong basic mechanism was targeted.

One important difference between the successful inhibitory effect of agents in animal models and the failure of the same therapies in man was the difference in dose that can be used.

It has become clear that for safety reasons it is not possible to give systemically in man the effective doses that may be required to inhibit the restenotic process. This led to the concept of local drug delivery. Local drug delivery with specially adapted balloon catheters, was hampered by a number of shortcomings. Delivery efficiency was low, retention of agent was poor since there was no targeting of agent to the vessel wall and the special delivery catheters could induce further vessel wall injury and required a prolonged procedure. Few clinical trials were completed.[26,27]

Drug-eluting stents

Delivering drugs from the stent itself reflects the most elegant form of local drug delivery and clearly has a number of advantages. Theoretically the local concentration will be high with the dose required being less than would be needed systemically, thus reducing the incidence of systemic side-effects. The agent is delivered to the site of need and can be tailored to the pathological process (to reduce thrombosis or restenosis in high risk cases). Retention difficulties can be overcome if the agent can be attached to the stent but then be made to elute off slowly once the stent is deployed. Achieving the correct balance between rate of elution and degree of retention is clearly important. Efficient ways of attaching the chosen agent to the stent are required.

Polymer coatings have been the subject of much discussion as they can themselves be responsible for local inflammation and neointimal proliferation.[28] The choice of the coating is therefore as important as that of the agent adsorbed to it. Ideally the agent should be applied to the stent directly with no polymer involved.

The following are prerequisites for stent-based local drug delivery to become clinically valuable.

The drug/agent should have the following characteristics:

- It should be effective, and because it is localized it can be potent.
- It should be able to target the cell type responsible for the pathobiological process preferentially.
- It should be effective when administered locally.
- It should bind to the stent/polymer and elute off into inter-strut vessel wall spaces.
- It should have known risks and side effects.
- Available data should enable an understanding of pharmacokinetic and dosing issues.

288

The stent should have the following characteristics:

- It should be as user friendly as current stents.
- It should be as safe and have the same longer term benefits (create large lumen, have good radial strength).
- It should not contribute to the restenotic process by inducing an inflammatory response. Thus if the drug-stent combination requires a polymer coating this polymer should be non inflammatory.

The following should be available for the stent/drug combination:

- Animal data demonstrating safety, pharmacokinetics, local cellular toxicity and, if possible, efficacy.
- Pilot studies initially testing safety.
- Longer term trials testing efficacy and safety.

Clearly, there are many targets for drug-eluting stent strategy, and they may be anti-inflammatory, antithrombotic and/or antiproliferative. Paclitaxel is an agent that has antiproliferative properties.

Paclitaxel and drug eluting stents

In 1963 an extract from the bark of *Taxus brevifolia*, a relatively rare plant was found to have cytotoxic activity against many tumours. It has specific properties against microtubules, promoting polymerization of tubulin, inhibiting the disassembly of microtubules, which thus become very stable and dysfunctional, and so inhibiting cell division.[29] Cell replication is inhibited in the G0/G1 and G2/M phases. Other effects include those on cell motility, shape and on transport between organelles. While it was recognized in the 1960s that the extract of the bark killed artificially preserved leukemia cells and was effective against advanced ovarian tumors, it was only in 1978 that it was shown that it killed cancer cells in a completely novel way by microtubular stabilization. However this property also causes side-effects by killing other rapidly dividing cells.

However, the first species used, *Taxus brevifolia*, had such low concentrations in the bark that the projected medicinal requirements would have destroyed the entire species within 10 years. Eventually paclitaxel has been produced through a semi-synthetic process.

Summary of the preclinical data

In vitro

- Hahnel *et al.*[30] assessed the effect of paclitaxel released by a biodegradable stent on vascular smooth muscle cells. The number of cells per high powered field was reduced by paclitaxel in a dose-dependent manner.

Exposure to 3.2 nmol or greater over 1 week resulted in a significant effect. Importantly, this was at local doses at least $10^5\times$ below systemic dosage.

- Voisard et al.[31] evaluated the effects of paclitaxel eluting from biodegradable stents on smooth muscle cells from human plaques. In combination with hirudin such paclitaxel-eluting stents reduced smooth muscle cell proliferation to 50% of controls (ranging from 55.5% to 61% reduction, depending on dose).

In vivo

The effect of paclitaxel has been tested in rat, rabbit and pig models with either local balloons or stents as delivery devices.

Rat model

- Kunert and colleagues[32] delivered 4 ml paclitaxel (10^{-5} mol/l) using a microporous balloon and showed a reduction in smooth muscle cell proliferation in both the intima and the media.
- Sollott et al.[33] extensively investigated the effects of paclitaxel on neointimal smooth muscle cell accumulation after angioplasty in the rat. The intimal medial ratio following balloon injury was 0.66 (0.08) for control but 0.18 (0.04) for paclitaxel treated vessels at 2 weeks ($P < 0.0001$).
- Farb et al. also investigated the effects in the rat carotid.[34] Stents containing 42 µg of paclitaxel had significantly less intima tissue formation in them (0.035 mm versus 0.06 mm control, $P = \leq 0.0001$).

Rabbit model

A number of authors have investigated the effects of paclitaxel on smooth muscle cell activity in the rabbit model.

- An important abstract was presented in 1998 in *Circulation* by Drachman et al.[35] The effects of paclitaxel-loaded stents were compared to polymer-coated and non-coated controls over 28 days. The neointimal area was reduced from 1.13 (0.13) mm^2 in uncoated controls to 0.29 (0.07) mm^2 in paclitaxel treated vessels ($P < 0.03$). Polymer-coated stents with no paclitaxel were similar to uncoated (1.28 (0.10)). The effect of paclitaxel loaded stents represented a reduction of 77% in intimal area. Positive remodelling was also demonstrated by this group.
- Similar benefits have been shown by others using balloon local drug delivery. For example, Herdeg and colleagues[36,37] using a rabbit model, showed that in paclitaxel-treated animals (double balloon to rabbit carotid

following electrically induced plaque) the intimal area increased only minimally from 0.179 mm^2 to 0.193 mm^2 at 8 weeks compared to an increase in the control animals to 0.301 mm^2. At 8 weeks positive remodelling (the opposite of the negative effects seen in man) was also evident (luminal area controls 0.417 mm^2: luminal area paclitaxel-treated 0.754 mm^2).

- Axel and co-workers[38] showed similar benefit in a rabbit artery injury model using a microporous balloon to deliver the paclitaxel. The mean intimal wall area at 28 days (0.21 (0.11)) was significantly less than controls (0.36 (0.29) $P = 0.01$, as was intimal thickness (110 (39) μm compared to 138 (85) μm in controls $P = 0.04$)). Interestingly, at the concentration used (10 μmol/l) endothelial regeneration was seen at the 28 day time period and was no different to controls. In this paper the in vivo benefits demonstrated were supported by in vitro findings of dose-dependent smooth muscle cell inhibition.

Porcine experiments

- In a pig coronary model, Kornowski et al.[39] from the Washington group, showed that a paclitaxel loaded stent (a Cook Corp. gRII) (dose = 175–200 μg/stent, with release in vitro kinetics of 0.75 μg/day for 30 days) deployed in the coronary artery resulted in a significant reduction in neointimal thickness (from 669 (357) μm in controls to 403 (197) μm in treated animals ($P < 0.05$)). Restenosis was reduced by about 50% (from 51 (27)% to 27 (27)%, $P < 0.05$). While the dose delivered was larger than was planned to be used in the clinical trial there is evidence that balloon pre-dilatation before stenting increases the injury index and thus increases the proliferative activity of the cells, making them potentially more sensitive to the agent.
- Heldman et al.[40] from the National Institute of Health in the USA, deployed paclitaxel-eluting stents into the carotid artery of rats. The doses used were 15 μg /stent and 90 μg /stent, similar to what is planned in man. Compared to controls the 90 μg/stent had a significant effect:

Paclitaxel dose (μg/stent)	Angiographic loss index	Histological neointimal area (mm2)
0	0.46 (0.04)	1.86 (0.25)
15	0.34 (0.07)	1.75 (0.21)
90	0.16 (0.06) (P < 0.003)	1.20 (0.13) (P < 0.05)

The combination of paclitaxel and the Cook Corp stent: porcine data

The data presented below are based on studies undertaken by Cook Incorporated. The purpose of the studies was to demonstrate safety. In general animal models are not standardized to reflect in-stent restenosis. There is thus ongoing concern about interpreting data from animal studies to determine the potential clinical efficacy. Thus initial animal work should comprise essentially safety studies and the clinical effectiveness of likely drug candidates be tested in pilot clinical trials. It is, however, important to understand what aspects of safety should be being assessed in the animal studies. Although the underlying mechanisms may be quite complex the safety endpoints for a coated stent in animal studies are relatively simple and include no increased mortality, no systemic toxicity, no increased thrombosis, no increase in restenosis and no aneurysm formation.

In three experiments compared to controls there was no excess neointimal response at 1 month (mm)

control 0.20 (0.12); 90 μg paclitaxel 0.12 (0.06)
control 0.24 (0.12); 90 μg paclitaxel 0.15 (0.08)
control 0.27 (0.13); 90 μg paclitaxel 0.22 (0.14)

nor at 6 months

control 0.16 (0.06); 90 μg paclitaxel 0.23 (0.08)

While these data do not show significant benefit they were not powered to do so, being safety data. In addition we know that part of the effect of paclitaxel on reducing recurrence after interventional procedures may relate to its positive remodelling, an effect similar to that seen with brachytherapy. Thus it is not surprising that an increase in vessel size was seen (control 2.79 ($\pm$0.11), 90 μg paclitaxel 3.17 ($\pm$0.34)), which in these studies may be the result of normal animal growth. Again the data presented were designed for safety not efficacy, but do show that at least the pigs treated with the highest dose stent did not show excess tissue formation and some positive remodelling. No aneuysm formation was seen. Re-endothelialization at the highest dose proposed for the clinical trial was approximately 75% complete at 1 month.

In other studies the amount of drug still on the stent at 14 days was 37%, demonstrating prolonged elution over time. In the doses to be tested in the clinical trial, no evidence of vessel wall haemorrhage, necrosis or significant inflammation was seen. No pigs suffered sudden death, suggesting in this sensitive model that thrombus was not an issue. The safety data from Cook are important because other pig studies of higher doses on different stent platforms have raised potential problems (Heldman, personal communication). Clearly stent platform, coating method and dose of paclitaxel may be critical.

All the stents tested (initially the GRII, then the V-FLEX stent) performed as per usual, with no delivery, track, pushablity or delivery problems. Sterilization undertaken at the time of production was not an issue and had no effect on drug efficacy, stability or release kinetics.

While other animal data (for example, from Frohlich's laboratory) indicated a U-shaped dose response with less benefit at higher doses, this was not the case with the Cook data, which demonstrated increasing benefit with increasing dose in the dose range tested.

There is little doubt that paclitaxel exerts strong effects locally on both smooth muscle cell activity and vessel wall dimensions after vascular injury. In three different animal models intimal thickness was reduced and positive remodelling has been shown. The clinical ELUTES (EvaLUation of Paclitaxel Eluting Stent) trial was devised around these studies. Important issues are:

- Re-endothelialization
- MACE at 6 months
- Longer term effects
- Efficacy and dose response

Ongoing trial – ELUTES

The ELUTES trial was planned primarily as a safety pilot with some markers of efficacy. A number off issues needed to be addressed:

- Prolonged antiplatelet medication To cover the potential for reduced re-endothelialization the period of antiplatelet medication was extended from the routine 1 month to 3 months.
- Positive remodelling Positive remodelling through an effect on medial/advential cell turnover/fibrosis is possible with agents such as paclitaxel, and is less likely in the stented patient because of the constraining influence of the stent. Longer term follow-up will include repeat angiography on those patients with any suggestion of increase in luminal diameter at first (6 month) quantitative angiographic measurement. This will be undertaken at 2 years.
- Animal data suggesting a U shaped curve. To address this issue the ELUTES trial is a dose finding study comparing four doses of paclitaxel (low, medium-low, medium, medium-high and high with control). It should be emphasized that high dose is approximately one-third of the dose shown by Frohlich's group to produce inflammatory changes in the pig model.
- Efficacy versus safety The primary endpoint for this trial is safety (MACE at 6 months). The trial is also powered to show a significant benefit in

diameter stenosis if one exists so this study will either remain a pilot study indicating a trend (or not) to enable the pivotal study to be appropriately powered or, if the differences reach significance, be the pivotal study.

The study

Study design

- Prospective, multicentre, randomized, triple blinded dose ranging with five treatment arms: control and four doses of paclitaxel.
- Stent platform: V-Flex Plus (3.0 or 3.5 × 16 mm),

Statistical calculations

- This study is powered at 80% to show a trend toward improvement in percent diameter stenosis from 35% to 25% ($P < 0.15$) for any one dose versus control.

To show this difference 180 patients are required in total (36 patients per treatment arm).

Primary endpoints:

- Effectiveness – %DS and late loss (by QCA) determined at 6 month follow-up by an independent angiographic core laboratory.
- Safety – major adverse cardiac events.

Steering committee:

Dr Anthony Gershlick, Glenfield Hospital UK (PI)
Dr Ivan De Scheerder, University Hospital Gasthuisberg
Dr Bernard Chevalier, Centre Cardiologique du Nord
Dr Alan Heldman, Johns Hopkins Medical Center
Dr Jeffrey Brinker, Johns Hopkins Medical Center

Important inclusion and exclusion criteria:

- Inclusion:
  Single lesion native vessel <15 mm length
  De novo lesion
  Reference vessel size 2.75–3.5 mm

294

Type A and B1 lesions
- Exclusion:
PCI in the setting of AMI
Contraindications to antiplatelet therapy

Current status of the ELUTES trial

The trial was completed in April 2001. The demographics to date indicate 84% male, 15% diabetics and 53% hypercholesterolaemic. The most stented artery has been the right, and most lesions (85%) have been types B1 and B2. To date there have been no medium term or late stent thromboses. The data will be reported in full in autumn 2001. There are likely to be further trials in the ELUTES series.

References

1. Moore RS, Rutty G, Underwood MJ et al. Time sequence of vessel wall changes in an experimental model of angioplasty. *J Pathol* 1994; **172**:287–92.

2. Carter AJ, Laird JR, Farb A et al. Morphological characteristics of lesion formation and time course of smooth muscle cell proliferation in a porcine proliferative restenosis model. *J Am Coll Cardiol* 1994; **24**:1398–405.

3. Waller B,F, Johnson DE, Schnitt SJ et al. Histologic analysis of directional coronary atherectomy samples. A review of findings and their clinical relevance. *Am J Cardiol* 1993; **72**:80E-87E.

4. Grant MB, Wargovich TJ, Ellis EA et al. Expression of IGF-I, IGF-I receptor and IGF binding proteins-1, -2, -3, -4 and -5 in human atherectomy specimens. *Regul Pept* 1996; **67**:137–44.

5. Marmur JD, Poon M, Rossikhina M Taubman MB. Induction of PDGF-responsive genes in vascular smooth muscle. Implications for the early response to vessel injury. *Circulation* 1992; **86**(Suppl 6):III53–60.

6. Strauss BH, Robinson R, Batchelor WB et al. In vivo collagen turnover following experimental balloon angioplasty injury and the role of matrix metalloproteinases. *Circ Res* 1996; **79**:541–50.

7. Topol EJ, Califf RM, Weisman HF et al. Randomised trial of coronary intervention with antibody against IIb/IIIa integrin for reduction of clinical restenosis: results at six months. *Lancet* 1994;**343**:881–6.

8. Mintz GS, Popma JJ, Hong MK et al. Intravascular ultrasound to discern device-specific effects and mechanisms of restenosis. *Am J Cardiol* 1996; **78**:18–22.

9. Carter AJ, Laird JR, Kufs WM et al. Coronary stenting with a novel stainless

steel balloon-expandable stent: determinants of neointimal formation and changes in arterial geometry after placement in an atherosclerotic model. *J Am Coll Cardiol* 1996; **27**:1270–7.

10. Serruys PW, de Jaegere P, Kiemeneij F *et al*. For the Benestent group. A comparison of balloon-expandable-stent implantation with balloon angioplasty in patients with coronary artery disease. *N Engl J Med* 1994;**331**:489–95.

11. Fischman D, Leon M, Baim D *et al*. A randomised comparison of coronary-stent placement and balloon angioplasty in the treatment of coronary artery disease. *N Engl J Med* 1994;**331**:496–501.

12. Klugherz BD, deAngelo DL, Kim BK *et al*. Three year follow up after Palmaz-Schatz stenting. *J Am Coll Cardiol* 1996; **27**:1185–91.

13. Eeckhout E, van Melle G, Stauffer JC *et al*. Can early closure and restenosis after endoluminal stenting be predicted from clinical, procedural, and angiographic variables at the time of intervention? *Br Heart J* 1995; **74**:592–7.

14. Wong SC, Baim DS, Schatz RA *et al*. Immediate resukts and late outcomes after stent implantation in saphenous vein graft lesions: the multicenter US Palmaz-Schatz experience. *J Am Coll Cardiol* 1995; **26**:704–12.

15. Foley JB, Brown RI, Penn IM. Thrombosis and restenosis after stenting in failed angioplasty: comparison with elective stenting. *Am Heart J* 1994; **128**:12–20.

16. Nunes G, Pinto I, Matters L *et al*. Coronary stenting in vessels smaller than 3 mm is associated with higher restenosis rates. *Eur Heart J* 1996; **17**:173 (abstract).

17. Moscucci M, Piana RN, Kuntz RE. Effect of prior coronary restenosis on the risk of subsequent restenosis after stent placement or directional atherectomy. *Am J Cardiol* 1994; **73**:1147–53.

18. Van Belle E, Bauters C, Hubert E *et al*. Restenosis rates in diabetic patients: a comparison of stenting and balloon angioplasty in native coronary vessels. *Circulation* 1997; **96**:1454–60.

19. Lau KW, Ding ZP, Johan A *et al*. Midterm angiographic outcome of single-vessel intracoronary stent placement in diabetic versus non-diabetic patients: a matched comparative study. *Am Heart J* 1998; **136**:150–55.

20. Baim DS, Lavine MJ, Leon MB *et al*. Management of restenosis within the Palmaz-Schatz coronary artery stent (the US multicenter experience). *Am J Cardiol* 1993; **71**:364–6.

21. Costa MA, Sabat M, van der Giessen JW *et al*. Late coronary occlusion after intracoronary brachytherapy. *Circulation* 1999; **100**:789–92.

22. Clowes AW, Karnowski MJ. Suppression by heparin of smooth muscle cell proliferation in injured arteries. *Nature* 1977; **265**:625–6.

23. Brack MJ. Ray S. Chauhan A. Fox J *et al.* The Subcutaneous Heparin and Angioplasty Restenosis Prevention (SHARP) trial. Results of a multicenter randomized trial investigating the effects of high dose unfractionated heparin on angiographic restenosis and clinical outcome. *J Am Coll Cardiol* 1995; **26**:947–54.

24. Powell JS, Clozel, Muller RKM *et al.* Inhibitors of angiotensin-converting enzyme prevent myointimal proliferation after vascular injury. *Science* 1989; **245**:186–8.

25. Gellman J, Ezekowitz MD, Sarembock IJ *et al.* Effect of lovastatin on intimal hyperplasia after balloon angioplasty: a study in an atherosclerotic hypercholesterolaemic rabbit. *J Am Coll Cardiol* 1991; **17**:251–9.

26. Camenzind E, Kint PP DiMario C *et al.* Intra-coronary heparin delivery in humans: acute feasibility and long term results. *Circulation* 1995; **92**:2463–72.

27. Meneveau N, Schiele F, Grollier G *et al.* Local delivery of Nadroparin for the prevention of neointimal hyperplasia following stent implantation: results of the IMPRESS trial. *Eur Heart J* 2001; **21**:1767–75

28. Van der Giessen. Lincoff AM, Schwartz RS *et al.* Marked inflammatory sequelae to implantation of biodegradable and nonbiodegradable polymers in porcine coronary arteries [see comments]. *Circulation* 1996; **94**(7):1690–97.

29. Jordan MA, Tosos RJ, Wilson L. Mechanism of mitotic block and inhibition of cell proliferation by paclitaxel at low concentrations. *Proc Natl Acad Sci USA* 1993; **90**:9552–6.

30. Hahnel I, Alt E, Resch B *et al.* Local growth inhibitory effect of paclitaxel released by a biodegradable stent coating on vascular smooth muscle cells. *J Am Coll Cardiol* 1998; 1114–102 (abstract).

31. Voisard R, Alt E, Baur R *et al.* Paclitaxel-coated biodegradeable stents inhibit proliferative activity and severely damage cytoskeletal components of smooth muscle cells from human coronary plaque material in vitro. *Eur Heart J Suppl* 1998; abstract P2109.

32. Kunert W, Kuttner A, Herdeg C *et al.* Paclitaxel inhibits development of restenosis following experimental balloon angioplasty in the rabbit carotid artery. *Eur Heart J* 1996; **17**:1998 (abstract).

33. Sollott SJ, Cheng L Pauly RR. Paclitaxel inhibits neointimal smooth muscle cell accumulation after angioplasty in the rat. *J Clin Invest* 1995; **95**:1869–76.

34. Farb A, Heller PF, Carter AJ. Paclitaxel polymer-coated stents reduce neointima. *Circulation* 1997; **96**:I-609 (abstract 3394).

35. Drachman DE, Edelman ER, Kamath KR. Sustained stent-based delivery of paclitaxel arrests neointimal thickening and cell proliferation. *Circulation* 1998; **98**(17S):P7401.

36. Herdeg C, Blattner A, Oberhoff M. Local delivery of paclitaxel in the rabbit carotid artery results in reduced neointima formation and vessel enlargement. *Eur Heart J* 1997; **18**(Suppl):460 (abstract 2695).

37. Herdeg C, Oberhoff M, Baumbach A. Local application of paclitaxel with the double balloon catheter in the rabbit carotid artery. *J Am Coll Cardiol* 1997; (Suppl); abstract 1038–76.

38. Axel DI, Kunert W, Goggelmann C. Paclitaxel inhibits arterial smooth muscle cell proliferation and migration in vitro and in vivo using local drug delivery. *Circulation* 1997; **96**:636–45.

39. Kornowski R, Hong MK, Ragheb AO. Slow-release paclitaxel coated GRII stents reduce neointima formation in a porcine coronary in-stent restenosis model.

40. Heldman IW, Hopkins J, Cheng L. Paclitaxel applied directly to stents inhibits neointimal growth without thrombotic complications in a porcine coronary artery model of restenosis. *Circulation* 1997; **96**(Suppl I):I–288 (abstract 1602).

36. THE BIOCOMPATIBLES' DRUG-ELUTING STENTS

Martin T Rothman and Andrew L Lewis

Stent drug delivery enables a drug to be delivered directly from a stent, targeting tissue more precisely than is possible with parenteral delivery. This allows the local administration of a therapeutic dose, increasing efficacy and reducing the risk of undesirable systemic side-effects.

The restenosis matrix

Restenosis is a complex multifaceted condition that consists of a number of phases.[1] Each of these events is a potential biological target that may enable control of the condition by administration of an appropriate pharmacologically active agent. It is unlikely that any one drug will be the answer to the restenosis problem in every patient type.

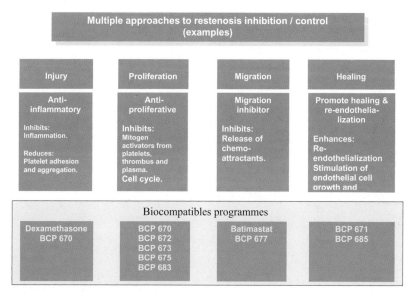

Figure 36.1: The restenosis matrix.

Biocompatibles' strategy is to build upon its unique coatings expertise to develop systems capable of delivering a range of compounds. Using this platform, one or more phases of the restenosis matrix may be targeted (Figure 36.1). This gives physicians the opportunity to select the most appropriate treatment for the patient from a broad range of therapeutic options.

PC Technology™ – the platform for drug delivery

Biocompatibles' proprietary coating, PC (phosphorylcholine) Technology is well suited to stent-mediated drug delivery because PC coatings are:

- Non-thrombogenic[2]
- Non-inflammatory[3]
- Compatible with critical stent mechanics
- Crosslinked for *in vivo* durability and stability

Biocompatibles has modified the PC coating, increasing the thickness of the coating on the outer (tissue) side of the stent, in order to maximize delivery of the compound to the vessel wall while minimizing systemic loss (Figure 36.2).

This modified proprietary coating has the ability to absorb and release a wide range of drugs safely and effectively, bringing the power of targeted drug delivery to interventional cardiology. This is achieved without compromising the crossing profile of the Bio*div*Ysio® stent.

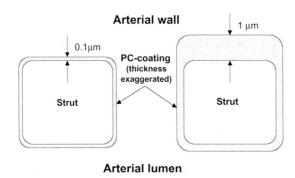

Figure 36.2: Bio*div*Ysio stent coating configurations (artist impressions).

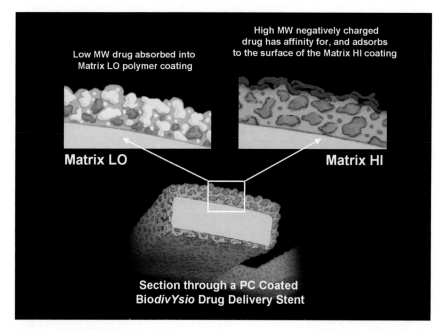

Figure 36.3: *Mechanisms of loading for BiodivYsio Matrix stents (artist impressions).*

BiodivYsio Matrix stents

There are two PC-coated drug delivery coronary stent formats currently available:

BiodivYsio Matrix LO stents with a coating especially designed to absorb and deliver drugs that are soluble in either an aqueous or organic solvent, with a molecular weight less than 1200 daltons.

BiodivYsio Matrix HI stents with a coating especially adept at interacting with negatively charged components found in many large biological molecules such as DNA, heparin, and oligonucleotides. It will easily adsorb and deliver compounds of molecular weight greater than 1200 daltons (Figure 36.3).

These BiodivYsio Matrix stents may be loaded with a variety of compounds by simply immersing them in a solution of a drug at the appropriate concentration for a few minutes. Once the stent is in place, the drug will be delivered to the target site over time. This self-loading approach allows physicians to select the most appropriate therapy for their patients.

301

Bio*divYsio* Matrix **LO** stents – technical specifications

Balloon diameters:	2.0, 2.5, 3.0, 3.5, 4.0 mm
Stent lengths:	10, 11, 15, 18, 28 mm
Recommended deployment pressure:	8 atm
RBP:	16 atm
¼ sizing:	14 atm
Crossing profile:	0.029 inch–0.047 inch
Guide catheter:	6 Fr

Bio*divYsio* Matrix **HI** stents – technical specifications

Balloon diameters:	3.0, 3.5, 4.0 mm
Stent lengths:	11, 15, 18, 28 mm
Recommended deployment pressure:	8 atm
RBP:	16 atm
¼ sizing:	14 atm
Crossing profile:	0.040 inch–0.047 inch
Guide catheter:	6 Fr

In vitro assessment

Drug loading

The swelling properties of the PC coating have been fully characterized by spectroscopic ellipsometry and neutron diffraction. These tests demonstrate that the majority of the coating hydrates within minutes of being placed within an aqueous environment.[5] This process is even faster in more effective solvents such as lower alcohols. Therefore, immersing the stent in an appropriate solution for just 5 minutes can lead to loading of a significant amount of compound.

The Bio*divYsio* Matrix stent coatings are capable of loading compounds of varying molecular weights and solubilities. The extent of loading is mainly controlled by the concentration of the loading solution in which it is placed (Table 36.1).

302

Table 36.1. Example drugs and their loading profiles on the BiodivYsio Matrix LO stent

Drug	Mode of action	Molecular weight	Loading example 1		Loading example 2	
			Loading concentration (mg/ml)	Amount on stent ($\mu g/cm^2$)	Loading concentration (mg/ml)	Amount on stent ($\mu g/cm^2$)
Dexamethasone	Anti-inflammatory	390	5	25	15	90
BCP682	Anti-proliferative	850	3	75	6	100
Batimastat	Anti-migratory	480	3	18	6	30
Angiopeptin	Growth factor inhibitor	1150	1	10	2	30

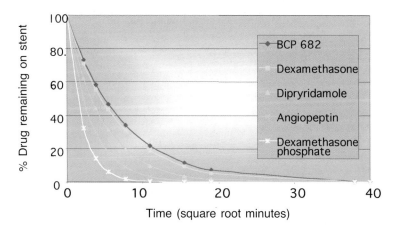

Figure 36.4: *In vitro release from* Bio*divYsio Matrix LO for a variety of compounds.*

Drug release

In-vitro studies investigating the release of the selected drugs from Bio*divYsio* Matrix drug delivery stents indicate essentially exponential decay release profiles (Figure 36.4). This is somewhat of a reflection of the drugs solubility profile in aqueous media, but also evidence of interaction with domains within the polymer for the more hydrophobic compounds.[6] This affords additional flexibility for tailoring release profiles. Therefore, the more hydrophobic the drug, the longer the time of elution – *vice versa* for hydrophilic compounds.

These results demonstrate the ability of PC Technology to release, in a controlled and sustained manner, a range of different pharmaceutical compounds. For all drugs investigated to date, 100% of the loaded amount has been shown to be released. This confirms that PC coating is purely an inert matrix for drug delivery and no specific irreversible interactions exist between the polymer and drug.

Preclinical data

A number of preclinical studies, mainly in porcine models, have been performed with a range of drugs using the Bio*divYsio* Matrix systems. The following sections summarize some of the important findings of these studies.

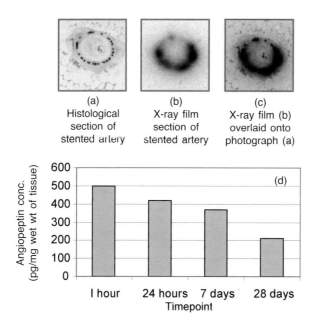

Figure 36.5: *Histology and autoradiography of an angiopeptin-loaded* BiodivYsio *Matrix LO stent.*

Site-specific and sustained delivery

Angiopeptin has been used previously in studies investigating treatments for restenosis, but as yet not using stent-based delivery. This relatively water-soluble compound was seen to elute fairly rapidly when assessed *in vitro*.[6] The *in vivo* release of ^{125}I-radio-labeled angiopeptin from the BiodivYsio Matrix LO system was performed in a porcine coronary model to determine if it could be delivered successfully to the artery.[7] Targeted tissue delivery of the angiopeptin was demonstrated as being > 96% to the stented portion of the LAD. After 28 days it was impossible to separate the stent from the vessel. In order to determine the drug's distribution, autoradiography and stent cross-sectioning were used. The cross-sectioning showed the stent position within the vessel (Figure 36.5(a)), while the autoradiograph showed the distribution of angiopeptin (Figure 36.5(b)). By superimposing the two images, the local distribution of the radiolabeled compound in the stented section could be confirmed (Figure 36.5(c)). The drug could still be detected in the tissue at high concentrations at 28 days after implantation (Figure 36.5(d)).

After deployment of the stents, angiopeptin was detected in the blood at 1 and 24 hours but after 7 days the level was reduced to zero. The peak blood level of the drug was achieved after 1 hour (0.5 ng/ml). Angiopeptin was

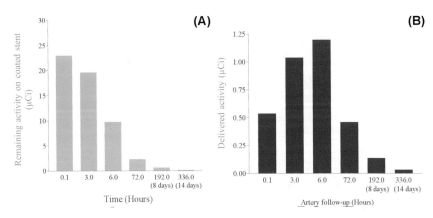

Figure 36.6: *Sustained release of DNA from a* BiodivYsio *Matrix HI drug delivery stent.*

detected in the urine at 1 hour (0.6 ng/ml) and at 28 days (0.2 ng/ml). Negligible amounts of the drug were detected in tissues outside the heart. These figures indicate the locality of angiopeptin delivery from the coated stent, demonstrating the very low systemic dose administered by this method.

Similarly encouraging results have been demonstrated by the delivery of ^{32}P-labeled 15 mer and 32 mer oligonucleotide sequences (4,700 and 10,000 molecular weight respectively, from the BiodivYsio Matrix HI platform (Figure 36.6).

Indications of efficacy for local drug delivery

The cortiocosteroids dexamethasone (DXM) and methylprednisolone (MP) were delivered locally from the BiodivYsio Matrix LO platform in a porcine injury model.[8] The histopathology and morphometric results shown in Table 36.2 relate to the acute inflammatory response and extent of neointimal hyperplasia at 5 days post-procedure. Both drugs are seen to decrease these adverse effects significantly.

Local delivery of an antimigratory compound, the matrix metalloproteinase inhibitor (MMPI) batimastat (British Biotech) has been studied using 18 mm BiodivYsio Matrix LO stents versus unloaded control stents. Vessel angiographic assessment before and immediately after stenting was compared with angiographic data after 1 month implantation. Neointimal area and

Table 36.2. 5-Day histopathological findings for corticosteroid delivery (see text for explanation)

Stent	Injury	Thrombus	Inflammatory response
Control	0.56 ± 0.27	0.74 ± 0.22	0.73 ± 0.22
DXM	0.40 ± 0.23	0.54 ± 0.23*	0.57 ± 0.20
MP	0.42 ± 0.18	0.50 ± 0.22*	0.51 ± 0.25*

(n = 12, *P <0.05 compared to control)

Stent	Lumen area (mm^2)	IEL area (mm^2)	EEL area (mm^2)	Neointimal hyperplasia (mm^2)	Area stenosis (%)
Control	7.94 ± 0.49	8.74 ± 0.44	10.44 ± 0.39	0.80 ± 0.16	9 ± 2
DXM	9.02 ± 0.49***	9.70 ± 0.49**	11.47 ± 0.69***	0.68 ± 0.12*	7 ± 1*
MP	8.35 ± 0.68	8.89 ± 0.73	10.26 ± 0.78	0.54 ± 0.16**	6 ± 2***

(n=12, * P <0.05, **P <0.01, ***P <0.001 compared to control)
DXM, dexamethasone; MP, methylprednisolone.

lumen size change were also compared between unloaded stents and stents loaded with batimastat (30 ± 7 µg/stent). Stents were implanted in a total of 24 vessels, with two different coronary arteries being selected using a balloon artery ratio of 1.15:1. Stents, 18 mm, were mounted on 3.5 mm diameter balloons and placed in vessels in the range 2.8–3.0 mm. Placement was controlled by IVUS with oversizing designed to induce injury and subsequent neointimal thickening; injury scores were similar for the control versus the group of stents loaded with batimastat. QCA showed lumen sizes of 2.3 mm for the control versus 2.8 mm for the drug-loaded stent at 28 days. As determined by histomorphometry, neointimal area showed a 40% decrease (P < 0.01) in the drug-loaded group (Figure 36.7).

Similar indicators of efficacy have also been observed when a proprietary drug from Abbott Laboratories was delivered from BiodivYsio Matrix LO stents. Using the same porcine model, reductions in neointimal thickness of 46% (P = 0.0001) and neointimal area of 43% (P = 0.008) and a corresponding increase in lumen area of 24% (P = 0.03) were reported. More recently, significantly increased MLD values were also obtained with BCP671 (a healing promoter, results not yet published).

These data are positive indicators for the efficacy of using drugs from each of the categories defined in the restenosis matrix, adding validity to the strategy as an approach to determining the best treatment options for the condition.

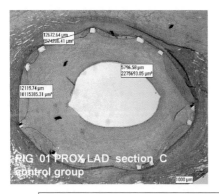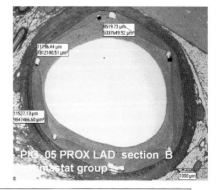

Measure	% Change	P value
Neointimal hyperplasia	−33	0.001
Lumen area	+15	ns

Figure 36.7: Histology from batimastat delivery from a BiodivYsio Matrix LO drug delivery stent at 28 days (Guy LeClerc, et al, unpublished data presented at local drug delivery meeting in Geneva 2001).

Clinical trials

Anti-inflammatory

Biocompatibles has recruited 71 patients into its first drug delivery clinical trial, the STudy of anti-Restenosis with BIodivYsio Matrix LO Dexamethasone Eluting stent (STRIDE), Principal Investigator, Ivan de Scheerder, Belgium. This is a multicentre prospective registry conducted in eight sites in Belgium. The study objectives were to evaluate the safety and efficacy of the BiodivYsio Matrix LO stent with dexamethasone, an anti-inflammatory drug. Patients will be evaluated at 1 and 6 months after stent implantation.

Anti-migratory

There is a clinical trial underway in Europe with a multicentre registry of 150 patients with de novo lesions, assessing the effectiveness of British Biotech's anti-migratory compound batimastat: Batimastat anti-Restenosis trIaL utiLIzing the BiodivYsio LocAl drug delivery PC steNT (BRILLIANT), Principal Investigators, Ivan de Scheerder, Belgium, and Bernard Chevalier,

France. This study will involve angiographic follow-up at 6 months and clinical follow-up at 1, 6 and 12 months.

Further studies with Bio*divYsio* stents preloaded with batimastat are planned throughout the world.

Others

Trials involving anti-proliferative and healing compounds are due to begin in 2001. In addition to company-sponsored trials, a number of therapeutic compounds are under assessment in physician-led clinical programmes around the world utilizing Bio*divYsio* Matrix stents for targeted drug delivery.

Future vision

Bio*divYsio* Matrix stents, with their capacity for drug delivery, offer the physician the opportunity for screening a variety of compounds with respect to their efficacy in the treatment of restenosis. In addition, data from clinical trials may help to determine whether there is a particular drug therapy best suited to different patient groups. Given the complexity of the restenosis process and variation in the response to stenting in humans, it is not unreasonable to expect that there may be a need for more than one therapeutic regime delivered via a stent from an appropriate polymer foundation.

Bio*divYsio* Matrix stents are not available in the USA.

References

1. Edelman E, Rogers C. Pathobiologic responses to stenting. *Am J Cardiol* 1998; **81**: 4E–6E.

2. Lewis AL. Phosphorylcholine-based polymers and their use in the prevention of biofouling. *Coll Surf B: Biointerfaces* 2000; **18**: 261–75.

3. Whelan DM, van der Giessen WJ, Krabbendam SC, *et al*. Biocompatibility of phosphorylcholine coated stents in normal porcine coronary arteries. *Heart* 2000; **83**: 338–45.

4. Lewis AL, Tolhurst LA, Stratford PW. Analysis of a phosphorylcholine-based polymer coating on a coronary stent pre- and post-implantation. *Biomaterials* (in press).

5.   Tang Y. Swelling of biocompatible polymer films. PhD Thesis, The University of Surrey, 2001.

6.   Lewis AL, Vick TA, Collias ACM *et al*. Phosphorylcholine-based polymer coatings for stent drug delivery. *J Mater Sci, Mater Medicine* (in press).

7.   Armstrong J, Gunn J, Holt CM *et al*. Local angiopeptin delivery from coronary stents in porcine coronary arteries. *Eur Heart J* 1999; **20**(Abst 366): 1929.

8.   De Scheerder I, Huang Y. Anti-inflammatory approach to restenosis. In: Rothman MT (Ed), *Restenosis: Multiple Strategies for Stent Drug Delivery (The Restenosis Matrix)*, ReMedica, 2001.

Trademarks

PC Technology and Bio*divYsio* are trademarks of Biocompatibles Ltd.

Patents

US Patents issued: US 5705583, US 5755771, US 6090901, US 6217608. Other patents pending.

37. The Boston Scientific Antiproliferative, Paclitaxel Eluting Stents (TAXUS)

Sigmund Silber and Eberhard Grube

Background and rationale

Restenosis in general, especially in-stent restenosis, is still the major limitation of percutaneous coronary interventions (PCI) and predominantly responsible for major adverse cardiac events (MACE) in follow-up studies and registries [Hoffmann and Mintz 2000]. Since in-stent restenosis is due to cell proliferation, stents coated with antiproliferative drugs promise to be the next revolution in the field of interventional cardiology [Gunn and Cumberland 1999]. The hope is that these drug-coated stents will overcome the problem of restenosis by providing lesion-directed intravascular delivery of drugs that interrupt the molecular cascade leading to in-stent restenosis. These drug-coated stents provide a perfect opportunity for local vascular drug delivery without prolonging the procedure. Potential advantages of drug-coated stents include:

a) targeted drug delivery to precise area requiring treatment
b) delivery at the time of implant injury
c) ongoing delivery through phases of healing
d) no additional materials or procedures required

Four interactive parameters may contribute to the success of a drug-coated stent in reducing restenosis: stent platform, selected drug(s), drug delivery vehicle or carrier, and the underlying vascular tissue. Stent implantation is associated with endovascular injury followed by a healing response. High degrees of injury appear to translate into more restenosis in the long term presumably because of more robust fibrotic healing responses. Ideally, the selected drug should interrupt multiple steps in the pathway that leads to restenosis, providing an effective anti-restenotic activity. For drug-eluting stents, the delivery vehicle must release the drug into the vessel in a manner that is consistent with the drug's mode of action. The drug and carrier must be compatible and together control drug release kinetics. Finally, the carrier and the drug individually or together have the potential to alter the tissue characteristics in the vessel. The cumulative effects of all these drug-coated stent parameters should interrupt the cascade associated with the healing response that culminates in restenosis.

The stent platform

The NIRx™ stent

The design of the NIRx™ stent is identical with the well-known stainless steel NIR™ stent (Figure 37.1). The NIRx™ stent is a premounted monorail (single operator exchange) system and combines the mechanical advantages of the NIR™ stent with a drug coating system (see below). Currently, the NIRx™ is available for clinical evaluation premounted on Boston Scientific's Advance catheter system (Figure 37.2). The distal section of the catheter has a dual lumen; the outer lumen is used for balloon inflation and the inner accepts a 0.014 inch guidewire. The Advance system is a monorail style stent delivery system (Figure 37.2). The proximal section is a single lumen stainless steel hypotube with a single luer port for inflation. The tip is tapered to facilitate advancement. The catheter will deliver 15 mm length stents with 3.0 mm and 3.5 mm diameter options. Only in TAXUS-I the stent had to be manually crimped.

Description of eluting coating

The carrier polymer encapsulating the NIR™ Conformer stent (Figure 37.1) is a proprietary formulation and impregnated with the antiproliferative drug paclitaxel (Figures 37.3 and 37.4).

The NIRx™ paclitaxel-coated stent uses a proprietary copolymer system as a carrier. Combining paclitaxel with the carrier system provides controlled release of the drug into the vessel wall. The technical development has included assessment of the effects of copolymer carrier system with and without various dose formulations of paclitaxel at various times in porcine stent implantation models. These studies have identified and refined the safe dose ranges for human trials and have provided insight into how paclitaxel alters the post-implant injury responses. The copolymer carrier system has been developed to provide homogeneous coverage of the stent platform after deployment (Figure 37.3) and deliver reproducible amounts of paclitaxel to the target area in the vessel. The carrier polymer is inert without effects on vascular healing up to 6 months after implantation [Rogers *et al* 2000]. The 15 mm NIRx™ stent holds 85 µg or 171 µg paclitaxel.

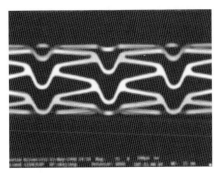 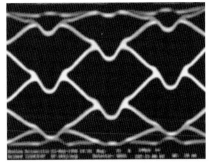

Figure 37.1: *The NIR™ Conformer stent: Geometry before (left) and after (right) expansion.*

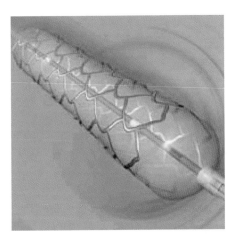

Figure 37.2: *The Advance catheter delivery system for the NIR™ and NIRx™ Conformer stent.*

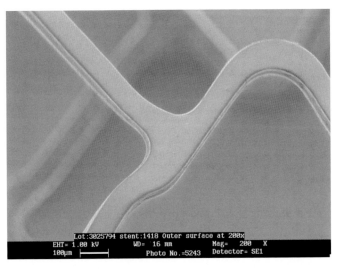

Figure 37.3: *Electron microscopic view of the expanded NIRx™ Stent (with coating).*

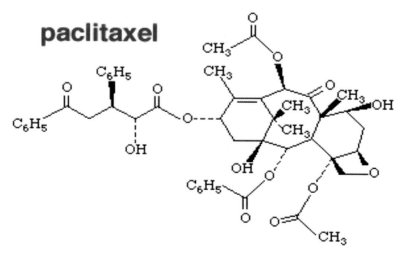

Figure 37.4: *Structural formula of paclitaxel. It was originally isolated from the bark of the Pacific Yew. It is a diterpenoid with a characteristic taxane-skeleton of 20 carbon atoms and has a molecular weight of 853.9 Daltons [Herdeg et al. 1998].*

Molecular action of drug

Paclitaxel is a trace compound found in the bark of the pacific yew tree in the northwestern USA (*Taxus brevifolia*). Today, synthetically produced Taxol® (Figure 37.4) has become a standard medication in oncology.

The antitumor activity of paclitaxel has been documented in vitro and in vivo. In 1992 the FDA approved it for solid tumors and in 1993 for ovarian cancer [Kristensen *et al.*, 1997]. Paclitaxel specifically inhibits microtubules by inhibiting their depolymerization resulting in an inhibition of cellular replication at the G0/G1 and G1/M phases [Wu *et al* 2001]. Paclitaxel exerts its pharmacological effects through formation of numerous decentralized and unorganized microtubules [Schiff *et al* 1979, Rowinsky *et al* 1995]. Substantial experience has been gathered with paclitaxel as it is the active ingredient in Taxol[11] (Bristol Myers Squibb). For chemotherapeutic purposes, it is administered systemically at concentrations greater than 3,000 fold higher than are being used for local stent delivery. Due to its specific inhibition of microtubules, it offers promise in preventing restenosis, stopping inflammation mediators and interrupting cell migration and proliferation [Sollott *et al* 1995, Axel *et al* 1997].

314

Elution profile

Paclitaxel interacts with arterial tissue elements as it moves under the forces of diffusion and convection and can establish substantial partitioning and spatial gradients across the tissue [Creel et al 2000].

In a bilateral rabbit iliac model two types of coated stents were investigated: the 7 cell/9 mm length containing 200 µg paclitaxel/stent (4.09 µg/mm^2, fast release, FR) or 50 µg paclitaxel/stent (1.02 µg/mm^2, slow release, SR). At day 1, the FR released approximately 70 µg and the SR appr. 2.4 µg. At the time of writing, the exact dose and release rates of the drug to be tested in humans based on preclinical in vivo and in vitro studies, will likely fall between 1.0 µg/mm^2 and 2.0 µg/mm^2 (loaded drug/stent surface area). For clinical studies, the SR stent will probably be as described above with 7 cell/15 mm containing 1.02 µg/mm^2 and therefore a total dose of 85 µg/stent. The FR will probably contain 2.04 µg/mm^2 and therefore a total dose of 171 µg/stent. Higher doses delivered in a sustained fashion seem likely to offer the best trade off between safety and efficacy [Rogers et al 2000].

Preclinical data

In vitro and in vivo data show that paclitaxel inhibits smooth muscle cell proliferation and migration in a dose-dependent manner in monocultures and co-cultures even in the presence of mitogens. The long-lasting effect after just several minutes' exposure time made this lipophilic substance a promising candidate for local antiproliferative therapy of restenosis [Axel et al 1997]. Local delivery of paclitaxel resulted in reduced neointimal stenosis and enlargement in vessel size. Both these effects contributed to a preservation of vessel shape and were likely to be caused by a structural alteration of the cytoskeleton [Herdeg et al 2000]. In rat carotid arteries, perivascular slow release of paclitaxel totally inhibited intimal hyperplasia [Signore et al 2001]. In a porcine model, paclitaxel-coated coronary stents produced a significant dose-dependent inhibition of neointimal hyperplasia in the LAD 28 days after implantation [Heldman et al 2001]. Delivery of paclitaxel into the intrapericardial space significantly reduced vessel narrowing in a balloon-overstretch model. This effect was mediated by a reduction of neointimal mass as well as a positive vascular remodeling [Hou et al 2000]. In the rabbit, neointimal hyperplasia is abolished for months after stent implantation, long after completion of drug delivery and polymer degradation [Drachman et al 2001].

Clinical data

The goals in the first human use feasibility studies in Europe are divided into two stages: first to evaluate safety of the triblock copolymer carrier system with low dose formulations of paclitaxel (TAXUS I). The second stage is an evaluation of two dose formulations of paclitaxel focusing on safety and estimates of efficacy for pivotal studies (TAXUS II–IV).

TAXUS-I

Purpose of TAXUS-I was to evaluate safety & feasibility of low-dose paclitaxel in the treatment of de novo and restenotic lesions in a prospective, controlled, randomized and double-blind study. The coated stents tested were seven cells/15 mm length (either 3.0 or 3.5 mm diameter) containing 1 µg paclitaxel/mm^2 (85 µg/stent). The corresponding uncoated NIR™ stents served as control. Inclusion criteria were lesions $\geq 50\%$ and $\leq 99\%$ and ≤ 12 mm in length with a reference vessel diameter of ≥ 3.0 and ≤ 3.5 mm (visual estimate). Patients with a LV-EF $< 30\%$, an MI within the past 72 hours, in-stent restenosis and patients with another planned coronary intervention within 90 days after study procedure were excluded. Post-procedure, 75 mg q.d. clopidogrel or 250 mg b.i.d. ticlopidine in addition to ASA was prescribed for 6 months. IVUS was part of the protocol in all patients at procedure and at 6 months. Clinical follow-up is planned at 12 months and up to 5 years. Enrolment into TAXUS-I is now complete. Sixty-one patients have been included at three German sites with 31 active and 30 controls (40 in Siegburg, 13 in Munich 8 and in Trier). Data for 30-day MACE (still blinded) is summarized in Table 37.1. The 6-month data will be available by November 2001.

Upcoming clinical trials

With the NIRx™ stent, several more studies have been initiated or are being planned:

TAXUS II

The primary objective of this study is to evaluate the safety and performance of the NIRx™ paclitaxel-coated stent compared with the uncoated NIR™ stent (PI: Antonio Colombo, Milan, Italy). Secondary objectives include

316

Table 37.1 TAXUS-1 study: MACE after 30 days (Grube, Silber and Hauptmann)

Event	Combined active and control arms
Death	0
Q-wave myocardial infarction	0
Target vessel revascularization	0
Stent thrombosis	0
Total	0

evaluation of MACE. In this multicenter, prospective, randomized and controlled study 532 patients should be enrolled in approximately 30 European centres. (133 patients randomized to NIRx™ and 133 to uncoated NIR™ control stent in each of the two cohorts = 4 × 133). In cohort 1, the slow-release formulation NIRx™ will be studied. If the safety profile is acceptable, the moderate-release formulation NIRx™ will be studied in cohort 2. All patients are to return for clinical follow-up 1 month and 6 months after stent placement. Telephone interviews are scheduled annually for 5 years. Angiography and intravascular ultrasound (IVUS) are required for all patients. The study is considered complete with regard to the primary endpoint after all patients have completed the 12-month follow-up.

Primary endpoint is the reduction of mean percent in-stent net volume obstruction at 6 months as measured by IVUS. Secondary endpoints are MACE as assessed 30 days, 6 and 12 months after stent placement and annually for 4 more years (i.e. 5 years after stent placement) and target lesion revascularization (TLR) as well as target vessel revascularization (TVR). Binary angiographic restenosis after 6 months is also considered a secondary endpoint. Inclusion criteria are similar to TAXUS-I.

TAXUS-III will investigate patients with in-stent restenosis. Finally TAXUS IV will be the pivotal study focusing on the paclitaxel eluting EXPRESS stent.

Future aspects

The TAXUS studies are designed to explore safety and utility of the Boston Scientific paclitaxel eluting stent. These studies will address the hypothesis that low levels of paclitaxel can blunt the initial response to injury and therefore prevent restenosis while still allowing vascular healing with endothelialization. Antiproliferative stents have clear advantages over radiation therapy: there is

Table 37.2   Brachytherapy vs. antiproliferative stents: similarities regarding smooth muscle cell (SMC) inhibition, reduction of restenosis and differences of low dose effects

	Brachytherapy	Antiproliferative stents
SMC inhibition	++	++
Restenosis reduction	+ (ISR)	+ (de novo)
Late thrombosis	+	+
Effects of low dose	Negative	None
Easy access	–	+

no low-dose stimulation in injured coronary segments [Serruys *et al*, 2001] and — of course — handling is much easier (Table 37.2). Long-term results of the paclitaxel stents according to various dosages [Rogers *et al*, 2000] and the experience with other antiproliferative stents [Sousa *et al*, 2001] will define the ultimate role of antiproliferative stents in interventional cardiology.

References

1.   Axel DI, Kunert W, Göggelmann C, Oberhoff M, Herdeg C, Küttner A, Wild DH, Brehm BR, Riessen R, Köveker G, Karsch KR: Paclitaxel inhibits arterial smooth muscle cell proliferation and migration in vitro and in vivo using local drug delivery. *Circulation* 1997;**96**:636–45.

2.   Creel CJ, Lovich MA, Edelman ER. Arterial paclitaxel distribution and deposition. *Circ Res* 2000;**86**:879–84.

3.   Drachman DE, Edelman ER, Seifert P, Groothuis AR, Bornstein DA, Kamath KR, Palasis M, Yang D, Nott SH, Rogers C. Neointimal thickening after stent delivery of paclitaxel: change in composition and arrest of growth over six months. *J Am Coll Cardiol* 2000;**36**:2325–32.

4.   Grube E, Silber S, Hauptmann KE. TAXUS-I: prospective, randomized, double-blind comparison of NIRx™ stents coated with paclitaxel in a polymer carrier in de-novo coronary lesions compared with uncoated controls. *Circulation* (abstr.), in press.

5.   Gunn J, Cumberland D. Stent coatings and local drug delivery. *Eur Heart J* 1999;**20**:1693–700.

6. Heldman AW, Cheng L, Jenkins M, Heller PF, Kim DW, Ware Jr. M, Nater C, Hruban RH, Rezai B, Abella BS, Bunge KE, Kinsella JL, Sollott SJ, Lakatta EG, Brinker JA, Hunter WL, Froehlich JP. Paclitaxel stent coating inhibits neointimal hyperplasia at 4 weeks in a porcine model of coronary restenosis. *Circulation* 2001;**103**:2289–95.

7. Herdeg C, Oberhoff M, Karsch KR. Antiproliferative stent coatings: Taxol and related compounds. *Semin Intervent Cardiol* 1998;**3**:197–9.

8. Herdeg C, Oberhoff M, Baumbach A, Blattner A, Axel DI, Schröder S, Heinle H, Karsch KR: Local paclitaxel delivery for the prevention of restenosis: biological effects and efficacy in vivo. *J Am Coll Cardiol* 2000;**35**:1969–76.

9. Hoffmann R, Mintz GS. Coronary in-stent restenosis – predictors, treatment and prevention. *Eur Heart J* 2000;**21**:1739–49.

10. Hou D, Rogers PI, Toleikis PM, Hunter W, March KL. Intrapericardial paclitaxel delivery inhibits neointimal proliferation and promotes arterial enlargement after porcine coronary overstretch. *Circulation* 2000;**102**:1575–81.

11. Kristensen GB, Tope C. Epithelial ovarian carcinoma. *Lancet* 1997;**349**:113–17.

12. Rogers C, Groothuis A, Toegel G, Stejskal E, Kamath KR, Seifert P, Hesselberg S, Delaney R, Edelman ER. Paclitaxel release from inert polymer material-coated stents curtails coronary in-stent restenosis in pigs. *Circulation* 2000;**102**:II–566.

13. Rowinsky EK, Donehower RC. Paclitaxel (Taxol). *N Engl J Med* 1995;**332**:1004–14.

14. Schiff PB, Fant J, Horwitz SB. Promotion of microtubule assembly in vitro by Taxol. *Nature* 1979;**277**:665–7.

15. Signore PE, Machan LS, Jackson JK, Burt H, Bromley P, Wilson JE, McManus BM. Complete inhibition of intimal hyperplasia by perivascular delivery of paclitaxel in balloon-injured rat carotid arteries. *J Vasc Interv Radiol* 2001;**12**:79–88.

16. Sollott SJ, Cheng L, Pauly RR, Jenkins GM, Monticone RE, Kuzuya M, Froehlich JP, Crow MT, Lakatta EG, Rowinsky EK, Kinsella JL. Taxol inhibits neointimal smooth muscle cell accumulation after angioplasty in the rat. *J Clin Invest* 1995;**95**:1869–76.

17. Serruys PW, Sianos G, van der Giessen W, Bonnier J, Urban P, Wijns W, Benit E, Vandormael M, Dörr R, Disco C, Debbas N, Silber S. Intracoronary β-radiation to reduce restenosis after balloon angioplasty and stenting. The Beta Radiation In Europe (BRIE) study. submitted for publication (2001).

18. Sousa JE, Costa MA, Abizaid A, Abizaid AS, Feres F, Pinto IMF, Seixas AC, Staico R, Mattos LA, Sousa AGMR, Falotico R, Jaeger J, Popma JJ, Serruys PW. Lack of neointimal proliferation after implantation of sirolimus-coated stents in human coronary arteries. *Circulation* 2001;**103**:192–5.

19. Wu K, Leighton JA. Paclitaxel and cell division. *N Engl J Med* 2001;**344**:815.

38. THE MULTI-LINK TETRA D™ DRUG-ELUTING CORONARY STENT SYSTEM

Guidant, Santa Clara, CA, USA

Patrick W Serruys and Susan Veldhof

Description	• Drug-eluting stent
	• Balloon expandable stent
	• Tubular design
	• Multiple rings connected with multiple links

History	• European ACTION clinical trial in progress

Rationale

Restenosis is a complex biological process. The promise of drug-eluting stents is that the stent scaffolding is designed to mitigate the mechanical components of the restenotic process, while the drug coating attacks the underlying biological mechanisms of restenosis.

Device description

The Multi-Link TETRA D™ drug-eluting stent is a balloon expandable stent designed specifically for treating coronary vessels. It is a tubular 3-3-3 corrugated ring design with six crests and variable strut thickness designed to provide high flexibility, conformability and radial strength without compromising scaffolding (Figures 38.1 and 38.2).

S.T.E.P.™ Balloon Technology is incorporated to reduce the amount of excess balloon material outside the stent and minimize the chance for edge dissections.

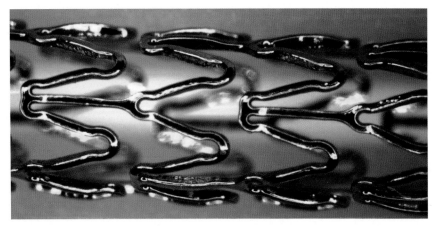

Figure 38.1: *Multi-Link TETRA D*™ *drug-eluting stent is a balloon-expandable stent with a tubular 3-3-3 corrugated ring design with six crests and variable thickness.*

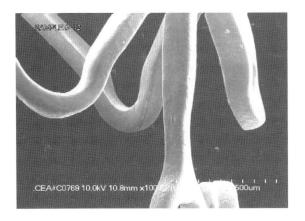

Figure 38.2:
Stent struts electropolished to a rounded smooth surface finish (SEM image, magnification 100×)

Multi-Link TETRA D™ drug-eluting stent offers low system profiles, modified GRIP™ Technology for stent security, proximal and distal balloon markers that indicate the position of the expanded stent and balloon working length and a lubricious hydrophilic coating to improve deliverability.

Multi-Link TETRA D™ stent technical specifications

Material composition:	316 L stainless steel
Degree of radiopacity (grade):	Moderate
Ferromagnetism:	Non-ferromagnetic (MRI safe)
Metallic surface area (expanded):	16% metal-to-artery ratio at 3.0 mm
Stent design:	Laser cut from a solid stainless steel tube in the corrugated ring pattern. Each ring is connected by 3-3-3 links
Strut design:	Unsupported surface area 3.4 mm^2 at 3.0 mm
Strut dimensions:	Thickness: variable thickness strut 0.0049–0.0036 inch
	Width: 0.0054–0.0032 inch
Longitudinal flexibility:	High
Percentage shortening on expansion:	4.3% (Family Average)
Degree of recoil (shape memory):	2.6% (Family Average)
Expansion range:	Maximum expansion 4.5 mm

Drug description

In the realm of interventional cardiology, prevention and reduction of neointimal hyperplasia are the most important requirements for a drug-eluting stent system. Actinomycin D has been tested extensively in the vascular arena of animal models to optimize the dose and release profile of the drug. Guidant has evaluated multiple dose release profiles for its drug-eluting stent in order to achieve an optimal vessel response. Evidence of re-endothelialization has been shown in the pre-clinical studies at the 28 day timepoint.

Actinomycin D is an antibiotic that has been approved for clinical use as an anti-cancer agent. The compound binds with DNA, preventing cell division and the production of proteins necessary for cell viability. Actinomycin D is cell cycle non-specific, meaning that cells in all phases of the cell proliferation cycle are affected by the drug. The performance of the drug is controlled by both the dosage (amount/concentration of drug on the stent), and release profile (the time period in which the drug elutes from the stent).

Actinomycin D is currently approved in most European countries and has been approved in the United States since 1964 with the indication for treatment of carcinoma of testis and uterus, Wilms Tumor, and other neoplasms.

Polymer description

The TRUE Coat™ (Targeted Release Uniform Elution) polymer is a bioinert coating on the stent that contains the drug (Actinomycin D). TRUE Coat™ is designed to control the release of Actinomycin D into the vessel wall over a period of time.

The TRUE Coat™ polymer must have long term compatibility. Guidant's preclinical studies have shown no adverse inflammatory, thrombotic, or neointimal responses at the 28 day (Figure 38.3) and 3 month time point.

The TRUE Coat™ polymer is designed to maintain its integrity through the manufacturing process, stent delivery, and stent deployment. Additionally, the TRUE Coat™ polymer membrane has the ability to be modified to alter the release rate of Actinomycin D over a given period of time. The flexibility of the TRUE Coat™ polymer was critical for the development of the Multi-Link TETRA D™ drug-eluting stent.

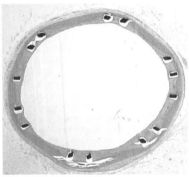

Figure 38.3: *Preclinical study showing no adverse inflammatory, thrombotic or neointimal response at 28 days.*

Preclinical testing

Guidant has performed numerous preclinical studies at acute and chronic endpoints utilizing multiple animal models. Significant inhibition of fibrocellular neointimal formation was observed with implantation of Actinomycin D eluting stents compared to control bare stents. Implantation of Multi-Link TETRA D™ drug-eluting stents at doses chosen for clinical study, were not associated with any adverse clinical symptoms. Pharmacokinetic studies performed with the Multi-Link TETRA D™ drug-coated stents demonstrated that local delivery of Actinomycin D to the vessel wall was obtained without evidence of systemic toxicity. Histopathology of multiple organs showed no indication of tissue toxicity at 7 days and 28 days after stent implant in the porcine model. In addition, presence of Actinomycin D was not detectable in the bloodstream after implant.

Preclinical studies to date have shown significant inhibition of neointimal proliferation and nearly complete endothelialization at the 1 month time point with the 2.5 µg/cm² and 10 µg/cm² doses (Figure 38.4).

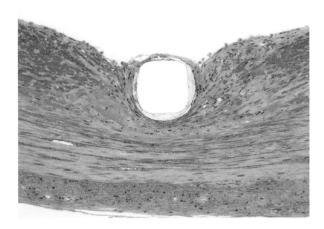

Figure 38.4:
Multi-link TETRA D™ 10 µg/cm² dose at 28 days.

Ongoing trials

Trial name:	ACTION clinical trial
Principal investigator:	Patrick Serruys
Number of sites:	Up to 30 sites from Europe, Australia, New Zealand, and South America
Number of patients:	360
Type of trial:	Randomized clinical trial
	Multi-Link TETRA coronary stent™ – control
	Multi-Link TETRA D™ drug-eluting stent – 2.5 µg/cm² dose
	Multi-Link TETRA D™ drug-eluting stent – 10 µg/cm² dose
Current status:	In progress

39. The Phytis DLC (Diamond-Like Carbon) Coated Stents

Phytis Medical Devices GmbH, Berlin, Germany

Norbert Sass, Gennady Fedosenko, Jürgen Hoge, Nico Margaris and Anastasios Salachas

Description	
	• The DLC coating on inner and outer surface consists of carbon atoms with saturated bonds and < 5% hydrogen.
	• The DLC coating is inert
	• The exceptional DLC-coating is bio- and haemocompatible thereby minimizing the multifactorial responses of the human body to foreign body implants
	• The smooth surface of DLC coated stents show increased adherence of human endothelial cells and a reduction of protein absorption and hence no denaturation
	• The DLC coating acts as a barrier for the heavy metal ions released from stainless steel
	• Very low elastic recoil, of 2.2%
	• Multicellular stent design with convex (Vario Wall™) expansion that starts in the middle of the stent and reduces risks of thorn and cutting trauma
	• Stents available as pre-mounted and bare version. Sizes: 9, 12, 16, 20, 25 mm and a side-branch stent (pre-mounted).

History	
	• 1996 Starting with research on different surfaces with biological considerations
	• End of 1996 : Selection of DLC coating
	• End of 1997 CE-Mark for the first generation of Phytis DLC stents
	• 1997 Foundation of the company Phytis
	• 1998 International distribution in over 20 countries
	• 1999 Presentation of the first clinical trial in Marseille: TVR in de Novo lesions 3.7%
	• Reorganization of the company and refined second generation of stents
	• 2000: ISO 9001/EN46001 certification
	• Starting with the double blind, randomized trial with Dr Antonio Colombo, Milan
	• 2001 Headquarters in Berlin, Germany

Technical specifications

Material composition:	316 L Stainless-Steel with Diamond-Like Carbon (DLC) coating
Degree of radiopacity (grade):	Moderate
Ferromagnetism:	None
MRI:	Non-ferromagnetic (MRI safe)
Metallic surface area	expanded: 16–20%
	unexpanded: 35–37%
Metallic cross-sectional area:	–
Stent design:	Slotted tube with rounded edges and multiple curved links
Strut thickness:	0.08 ± 0.01 mm
Profile(s): non-expanded (uncrimped):	1.6 mm
on the balloons:	0.9–1.15 mm
Longitudinal flexibility:	Excellent
Percentage shortening on expansion:	Between 4.5 and 5.5% at 3.5 mm diameter
Expansion range:	2.0–5.5 mm
Degree of recoil (shape memory):	2.0–2.2%
Radial force:	High
Currently available diameters:	9, 12, 16, 20, 25 mm
Currently available lengths mounted/implanted:	9, 12, 16, 20, 25 and side-branch stent (17.7 mm)
unmounted:	9, 12, 16, 20
Currently available sizes:	From 2.5 to 4.0 mm
Recrossability of implanted stent:	Yes
Other non-coronary types available:	In development

Phytis DLC coated stent delivery system

Type of deployment system	Rapid-exchange hypo-tube delivery catheter
Balloon type	Semi-compliant, high pressure
Balloon material	Nylon based Co-polymer Blend
Nominal pressure	6 atm
Rated burst pressure	16 atm
Guide wi re lumen	0.014 inch (max)
Distal shaft size	2.7 Fr
Proximal shaft size	2.0 Fr
Recommended min. guiding catheter	6 Fr
Radiopaque markers	Proximal and distal to stent
Crimped profile of stent	1.0 1.1 mm (depending of balloon diameter)

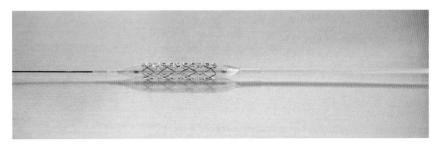

Figure 39.1: DLC-coated stent.

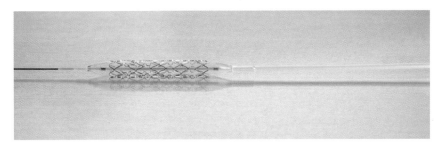

Figure 39.2: DLC-coated stent.

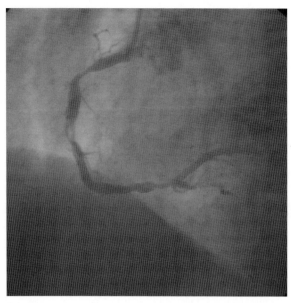

Figure 39.3:
(a) After 6 months;
(b) post-implantation;
(c) pre-implantation.

(a)

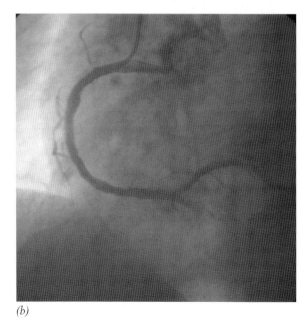

(b)

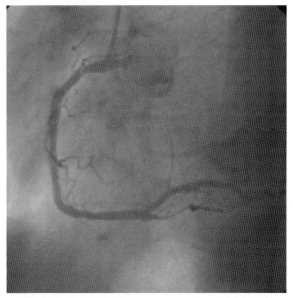

(c)

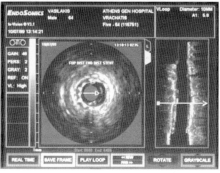

(a)

Figure 39.4: *IVUS pictures at 6 months follow-up.*
(a) No restenosis. There was very little accumulation of fibrous material.
(b) The reduction in MLD at the 6 months follow-up compared with the time of implantation was less than 10%. (Courtesy of Dr Vrachatis, Athens, Greece.)

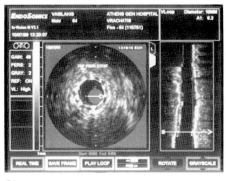

(b)

Tips and tricks

It is important to know that the Phytis Diamond stent in contrast to bare stainless steel stents is suitable for allergic patients, even if they are allergic to heavy metal ions.

Ongoing trials

Name	Purpose	Number of patients	Principal investigator	Centres	Design
DRASTIC	Coated versus Uncoated stents	380	Dr A. Colombo	4	Double blind, randomized
HEDIM	Clinical versus QCA restenosis	240	Dr A. Tavernarakis	3	Randomized
DOSIS	Clinical follow up of MACE	600	Dr J. Ubago	25	Open registry
ORCHIDS	Primary versus pre-dilatation	240	Prof. Huo/Prof. Ge	14	Randomized
MATIS	Metal allergy	230		2	Randomized

Indications for use

- De Novo coronary lesions (primary employment in case of stenosis or closures)
- Restenosis after PTCA
- Vein bypass stenosis or closure
- High risk of restenosis after PTCA
- Dissection after PTCA
- Recoil after PTCA
- Acute vascular occlusion
- Sub-optimal result after PTCA

THE PHYTIS DLC (DIAMOND-LIKE CARBON) COATED STENTS

Why I like my stent

The unique qualities of the Phytis Diamond Like Carbon coated stents are the result of a development process that did not start from the technical side, but with biological considerations. From the early beginning of the research and development process the stent was designed to prevent restenosis. From the moment the first study results were published it was clear, that the concept, to minimize restenosis by an inert, protecting and thrombo-resistent extremely smooth and durable coating, was correct. Biocompatibility was the keyword to clinical success in the Diamond stent concept.

1. The Phytis Diamond Like Carbon coated stent has the lowest restenosis rate reported (3.2%–4.1%).
2. It is the only stent coating that is able to protect the surrounding tissue from all negative side effects of the stainless steel, such as toxic and allergic reactions from heavy metal ions, adhesion of platelets and activation of the immunological cascade.
3. The DLC-coating remains intact after dilatation and more than 400,000,000 heartbeats without a scratch or breaking under the electron microscope.
4. It's anti-allergic effects and its flexible structure make the DLC-coating unique in comparison to other coatings.
5. Allergy to stainless steel is a contraindication for using uncoated L316 stainless steel stents. Due to the total inhibition of heavy metal ion release no prior allergy diagnosis is necessary for using the Phytis DLC-coated stents.

Clinical trials

Köster et al (2000) investigated whether in-stent restenosis might be triggered by contact allergy to heavy metal ions from 316 L stainless-steel stents by percutaneus allergy testing and QCA (quantitative coronary angiography).

It was found that all patients with specific positive allergy test results also had in-stent restenosis from 50% to over 70% after 1–6 months. All of these patients had recurrent angina pectoris and needed TLR.

Also non-specific irritant reaction in the patch test lead to a higher restenosis rate than in the patient group without allergy test reaction.

It was emphasized that stainless steel implants can cause inflammatory hypersensitivity reactions and allergic reactions to metal, which lead to a fibroproliferative response around the implant.

Barragan (1999) – the Paul Barrragan single centre study with 6–month clinical follow up was presented in Marseilles. A total of 250 De Novo Lesions treated in 165 patients, with a clinical TLR of only 3.7%.

Gutensohn et al (2000) examined the reduction of metal ion release, platelet activation and thrombogenicity by diamond-like carbon coated stents in comparison to 316 L stainless steel stents. There were high concentrations of molybdenum and nickel released from non-coated stents, whereas metal-ion release from DLC-coated stents was virtually undetectable. The concentrations of CD62p and CD63, which indicate platelet activation was significantly higher in non-coated stents.

His conclusion is, that diamond-like coated stents significantly improves biocompatibility and therefore reduces thrombogenicity

Margaris (1998) implanted the DLC-coated stents into 105 De Novo Lesions at 97 patients. Clinical restenosis defined as recurrence of angina or positive stress test in the three months follow up was obtained in only four cases. Not in a single case of TLR was necessary.

Salachas (2001): treated 96 patients with 121 De Novo Lesions with 128 Phytis DLC-coated stents, followed by a thallium scan test after 6 months. Only nine patients showed a positive result: five patients suffered from in-stent restenosis; four patients showed lesion progression elsewhere. The overall angiographic restenosis rate was only 4.1%.

References

1. Köster R, Vieluf D, Kiehn M, Sommerauer M, Kähler J, Baldus S, Meinertz T, Hamm CW. Nickel and molybdenum contact allergies in patients with coronary in-stent restenosis. *The Lancet* 2000;**356**:1895–7.

2. Gutensohn K, Beythien C, Bau J, Fenner T, Grewe P, Koester R, Padmanaban K, Kuehnl P. In vitro analyses of diamond-like carbo coated stents. Reduction of metal ion release, platelet activation and thrombogenicity. *Thromb Res* 2000;**99**:577–85.

3. Margaris N, Salachas A, Tsakliadou I, Tsilias K, Antonellis I, Ifantis G, Efremidis M, Prappa E, Philippatos G, Kanatsellos C, Tavernarakis A. Intracoronary Phytis DLC stent implantation without subsequent anticoagulation or intravascular ultrasound guidance. Experience from a single center. XXth Congress of the European Society of Cardiology, Vienna, Austria (1998).

4. Salachas A, Antonelis J, Margaris N, Ifantis G Tavernakis A. Intracoronary DLC Phytis stent implantation. Experience from a single center. The Paris Course on Revascularization (PCR) 2001.

5. Simeoni J B, Roquebert P O, Sainsous S, Bayet G, Silvestri M, Barragon P. Phytis stent registry. Endocoronary Biomechanics and Restenosis Symposium, Marseille 1999.

40. THE PHYTIS DOUBLE-COATED STENT

17-β-estradiol eluting polymer-coating in combination with the Phytis Diamond-Like Carbon coating

Phytis Medical Devices GmbH, Berlin, Germany

Norbert Sass, Holger Anhalt and Thomas Glandorf

Rationale

In-stent restenosis of about 25% after implantation of stainless steel stents is the major problem in PTCA procedures today. PTCA and the dilatation of the stent system means a severe trauma to the coronary artery wall. Wounds and fissures up to the media of the vessel wall are caused by high-pressure expansions of the balloon. The implantation of the foreign body (stent) and the vessel injury cause a complex immune reaction, with platelet and macrophage aggregation in the beginning and neointimal formation as the end result of the cascade.

The way to solve in-stent restenosis is to inhibit the process that leads to intimal hyperplasia after stenting, the reason for restenosis.

Neointimal thickening is caused by uncontrolled proliferation and migration of arterial Smooth Muscle Cells (SMC) into the lumen of the coronary vessel. The PTCA-procedure also causes denudation of the endothelial cell layer. Until this endothelial layer has been re-established the wound healing process remains unfinished.

The favourable characteristics of the Diamond Like Carbon Phytis Diamond-Like Carbon coated stent from Phytis have reduced the rate of in-stent restenosis to less than 5% in de novo lesions, the lowest rates reported.

The way to a further reduction of restenosis is the local application of drugs after stent implantation, the drug-eluting concept.

Description of the eluting coating

The eluting coating consists of several layers of a degradable polymer. When the polymer degrades, the drug that had been included in the polymer structure is released. By loading these polymer layers with different amounts of 17-β-estradiol it is possible to modulate the eluting curve exactly as wanted. When no more drug application from the eluting polymer is necessary after a couple of weeks, the coating has degraded completely and the unique properties of the underlying Phytis Diamond-Like Carbon (DLC) coating still protect the organism from the negative effects of stainless steel.

Molecular action of the drug

Recently the leading stent manufacturers for drug eluting stents have investigated several drugs. Although it has been possible to stop SMC-proliferation, the cytotoxic effects of these drugs inhibited re-endothelialization, which means antagonization of the wound healing process.

In contrast to that, several experimental studies have shown, that 17-β-estradiol not only inhibits the SMC-proliferation in a reversible, non-cytotoxic and dose dependent way, but it also leads to a significantly faster re-endotheliazation of the traumatized coronary vessel. These favourable pharmacological actions of the 17-β-estradiol are achieved due to a number of pharmaceutical actions of the drug, based on the receptor model and on direct effects to the cell membranes.

17-β-Estradiol has the ability to act in different ways on SMC and endothelial cells. It stops the unwanted mitogene process of SMCs activated by cytokines and activates on the other hand a wanted mitogen process in endothelial cells. This antagonistic action of the drug is achieved due to different concentrations of the two known receptors ER-alpha and ER-beta. ER-alpha is highly concentrated in SMCs, while ER-β is responsible for the genomic actions of the drug in endothelial cells.

The promotion of re-endotheliazation is, compared to other discussed drugs, a unique quality of 17-β-estradiol.

The 17-β-estradiol eluting double-coated stent concept unites the favourable characteristics of the Phytis Diamond-Like Carbon coating in terms of fast endothelial growths, inhibition of immune reaction and anti-allergic properties with the 17-β-estradiols ability of non-toxic inhibition of SMC-proliferation and migration and acceleration of re-endotheliazation of the denudated coronary wall. Therefore, this double-coating concept might enhance the wound healing process after coronary vessel injury with subsequent reduction of restenosis.

17-β-Estradiol pharmacodynamiques:

In therapeutic doses there are gender-independent and dose-dependent effects on SMC proliferation/migration and endothelial recovery. The effect is not a toxic one. After termination of medication, it has been proven that SMC are still able to proliferate.

338

Estradiol and SMC:

17-β-Estradiol effects SMC- proliferation/migration principally by genomic and nongenomic mechanisms.

Genomic effects:
- Gene expression by interacting with estrogen receptors (ER-alpha) and other transcription factors.

Non-genomic effects:
- Stimulates membrane mediators and second messengers
- Inhibits response on cytokine-triggered SMC-stimulation (for example: PDGF and bFGF)
- 17-β-Estradiol modulates the vascular inflammatory response by inhibiting cytokine activation and expression of adhesion molecules
- Induction of VEGF in epithelial cells and fibroblasts (VEGF inhibits SMC proliferation/migration of SMC and increases endothelial recovery by its mitogenic effect on endothelial cells)
- Inhibits platelet aggregation and platelet adhesion
- Decreases SMC proliferation/migration by inhibition of thymidine up-take.
- Direct effects on the vessel wall (ion-channels, especially modulation of calcium-influx and activation of membrane-proteins)
- Increase of NO-concentration inhibits SMC-proliferation/migration

Estradiol and endothelial cell recovery:

Mechanisms that are responsible for the promotion of endothelial recovery by 17-β-estradiol after denudation:

Genomic effect:
- mRNA transcription is enhanced by 17-β-estradiol modulated by endothelial cell specific estradiol receptors (ER-β)

Nongenomic effects:
- Increase of NO by 17-β-estradiol results in significantly faster re-endotheliazation
- 17-β-Estradiol induced VEGF and other angiogenetic growth factors promote fast endothelial recovery

In this context it is important to mention that several studies could prove that fast re-endotheliazation correlates inversely with formation of neointima formations.

Eluting profile

The local application of the drug is most important the first days after the trauma when all anti-inflammatory and vessel wall repair mechanisms are most active. Therefore in the first week the eluting rates are the highest. Then the polymer coating constantly elutes a low dose rate for a couple of weeks. Finally the wound healing process of the coronary vessel wall is finished and no more local drug application is necessary.

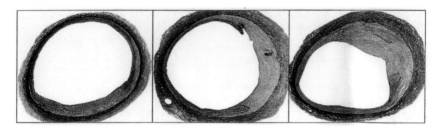

Figure 40.1: *Representative light micrographs ($\times 40$) of arterial segments from the three treatment groups: (A) BE-treated artery (extent of injury $= 0.23$, neointimal area $= 0.24$ mm^2); (B) PTCA only-treated artery (extent of injury $= 0.29$, neointimal area $= 1.00$ mm^2); and (C) vehicle only-treated artery (extent of injury $= 0.23$, neointimal area $= 1.3$ mm^2). Reproduced with permission from Chandasekar et al (2000).*

Preclinical data

a) In the latest Quebec-study Chandrasekar (2000) tested the local one-time application of 600 μg 17-β-estradiol directly after experimental stenting of juvenile farm pigs. The result was a markedly lower proliferative response than in the control group.

b) Finking et al (2000) showed a gender-independent inhibition of neointimal growths at a 17-β-estradiol concentration of 50 μg/ml in a rabbit-aorta cell cultural model. He emphasizes that the inhibitory effect is not toxic, but reversible after withdrawal of medication.

c) Somjen et al (1999) showed, that positive effect on re-establishing the endothelial layer of PD-ECGF (platelet-derived endothelial cell growth factor) was doubled by 17-β-estradiol. Many other publications demonstrated enhanced, receptor triggered, VEGF-expression by 17-β-estradiol.

d) Ashcroft et al (1999) examined the influence of topical 17-β-estradiol on cutaneous wound healing and came to the conclusion that 17-β-estradiol significantly diminished delays in wound healing, caused by a direct inhibition of neutrophile chemotaxis and down regulation of cell-adhesion molecules (l-selectin), which are important for the initiation of the immunologic cascade. The result was a strong reduction of neutrophils in the wound area and a significant reduction of wound-size. It was concluded that the inhibition of neutrophile response also leads to attenuation of neutrophile adherence to the coronary vascular endothelium. The same authors report a significantly accelerated wound healing compared to age-match controls.

Clinical data

First feasibility studies in human beings are planned for the beginning of 2002.

Upcoming clinical trials

In addition to the extensive amount of already published data concerning 17-β-estradiol animal trials will be carried out in the near future, to determine the best dose of the drug.

References

Ashcroft GS, Greenwell-Wild T, Horon MA *et al*. Topical estrogen accelerates cutaneous wound healing in aged humans associated with an altered inflammatory response. *Am J Pathol* 1999;**155**:1137–1146.

Bausero P, Ben-Mahdi M, Mazucatelli J *et al*. Vascular endothelial growth factor is modulated in vascular muscle cells by estradiol, tamoxifen, and hypoxia. *Am J Physiol Heart Circ Physiol* 2000;**279**:H2033–H2042.

Chandrasekar B, Tanguay JF. Local delivery of 17-Beta-Estradiol decreases neointimal hyperplasia after coronary angioplasty in a porcine model. *J Am Coll Cardiol* **36**:1972–8.

Chen SJ, Li H, Durand J *et al*. Estrogen reduces myointimal proliferation after injury of rat carotid artery. *Circulation* 1996;**93**:577–84.

Dai-Do D, Espinodg E, Liu G et al. 17β-estradiol inhibits proliferation and migration of human vascular smooth muscle cells: similar effects from postmenopausal females and in males. *Cardiovasc Res* 1996;**32**980–85.

Finking G, Leuz C, Wohlfrom M, Hanke H. In vitro Modell zur Untersuchung der Wirkung von Östrogenen auf die Neointimabildung nach Endothelverletzung an der Kaninchenaorta. *ALTEX* 2000;**17**:11–14.

Finking G, Walkenhauer M, Łeuz C, Hanke H. Post-injury ex vivo model to investigate effects and toxicity of pharmacological treatment in rings of rabbit aortic vessels. *ALTEX* 2000;**17**:67–74.

Gutensohn K, Beythien C, Bau J *et al*. In vitro analyses of diamond-like carbon coated stents. Reduction of metal ion release, platelet activation, and thrombogenicity. *Thromb Res* 2000;**99**:577–85.

Hanke H, Hanke S, Finking G *et al*. Different effects of estrogen and progesterone on experimental atherosclerosis in female versus male rabbits. Qualification of cellular proliferation by bromodeoxyuridine. *Circulation* 1996;**94**:175–81.

Karas RH, Hodgin JB, Known M *et al*. Estrogen inhibits the vascular injury response in estrogen receptor β-deficient female mice. *Proc Natl Acad Sci USA* 1999;**96**:15133–6.

Krasinski K, Spyridopoulos I, Asahara T *et al*. Estradiol accelerates functional endothelial recovery after arterial injury. *Circulation* 1997;**95**:1768–72.

Somjen D, Jaffe A, Knoll E *et al*. Platelet-derived endothelial cell growth factor inhibits DNA synthesis in vascular smooth muscle cells. *Am J Hypertens* 1999;**12**:882–9.

Vargas R, Vargas R, Wroblewska B *et al*. Oestradiol inhibits smooth muscle cell proliferation of pig coronary artery. *Br J Pharmacol* 1993;**109**:612–17.

Zancan V, Santagati S, Bolego C *et al*. 17β-Estradiol decreases nitric oxide synthase II synthesis in vascular smooth muscle cells. *Endocrinology* 1999;**140**:2004–9.

41. THE QUANAM QUADDS-QP2 STENT

Boston Scientific Corportion Inc/Quanam Medical, Santa Clara, CA, USA

Sigmund Silber, Eberhard Grube and Peter Fitzgerald

Background and rationale

The concept of delivering — or eluting — a drug from a stent over a period of time to treat the problem of in-stent restenosis following stent implantion is an attractive strategy. Local drug delivery for cardiovascular disease, prior to the advent of stents, was restricted to catheter-based delivery. These technologies were limited by the compounds available for catheter-based delivery, dwell time of the delivery catheter and length of residence time of these compounds in the vessel wall following completion of the delivery. Stent-based drug delivery offers a platform for not only maintaining compounds directly at the site of injury or disease and providing prolonged delivery, but it also allows for the delivery of hydrophobic compounds which cannot be easily delivered via conventional methods.

The stent platform

The QuaDDS-QP2 stent is based on the uncoated QueST stent platform (formerly Quanam Medical Corporation). The QueST stent is laser cut from one continuous piece of 316L stainless steel tubing and does not require subsequent welding or joining. The slotted tube stent is premounted on an over-the-wire polyethylene balloon. The QueST consists of individual segments, each 3.8 mm long, connected by inter-segment connecting links (Figure 41.1). The shaft of the delivery system is coaxial over the distal section and compatible with a 0.014 inch guidewire. The stent delivery system has two radiopaque (platinum) markers.

Description of eluting coating

The QuaDDS stent is a QueST stent covered with a series of 2 mm (width) polymer sleeves made from an acrylate polymer and formed into ringed sleeves (Figure 41.1). The sleeves have a thickness of approximately 0.0025 inch (half the thickness of a stent strut). The stent length determines the number of sleeves which are placed equidistant from each other over the length of the stent to prevent total stent coverage. For example, a 13 mm stent length would carry four sleeves. The non-biodegradable proprietary polymer sleeve is loaded with the microtubule stabilizer 7-hexanoyltaxol, also referred to as QP2. QP2 is loaded into the polymer sleeve by dissolving the drug into a solvent that absorbs into and swells the polymer. The polymer absorbs a specified volume of the solution at a known concentration. The solvent is subsequently removed by vacuum drying. The total dose per sleeve is approximately 800 µg. Therefore, the 13 mm stent carries 3.2 mg and the 17 mm stent a dose of approximately 4.0 mg of QP2.

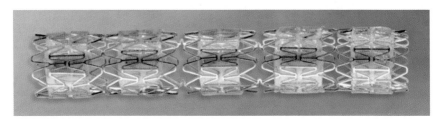

Figure 41.1: *The Quanam QueST stent consists of individual segments each 3.8 mm long joined by inter-segment connecting links. On the QuaDDS-QP2 stent a non-biodegradable proprietary polymer is ensheathing the QueST stent loaded with the slow-release microtubular inhibitor 7-hexanoyltaxol ('taxen').*

Molecular action of drug

Quanam has evaluated a number of drugs for their effectiveness in minimizing restenosis after stent placement in non-atherosclerotic rabbits and pigs. Of the drugs evaluated, paclitaxel showed a positive effect in reducing neointima. However, the desire to extend drug retention for a longer period of time than that of paclitaxel, the more hydrophobic derivative of paclitaxel, 7-hexanoyltaxol (QP2, called a 'taxen') became the focus of investigation [Kingston 1991]. The mechanism of activity is similar to that of paclitaxel, in that it inhibits microtubule formation by inhibiting microtuble depolymerization thus interferring in the cell cycle at the the G2/M phase. QP2 is about half as soluble as paclitaxel, which has a solubility of 1 µg/ml.

Elution profile

In vivo drug release studies in a rabbit iliac model have demonstrated that approximately 80% of QP2 is released within the first 90 days following a continuous sustained release profile with the drug still being released at 180 days. Tissue retention was maintained at a relatively constant level over a 90-day period with the drug being identified in arterial tissue at 180 days. The amount of QP2 either 1 cm proximal or distal from the stent edge was determined to be 1/10 to 1/100 of the amount found in the tissue within the stented segment. There was no detectable drug in the other tissues investigated. This indicates that under the experimental conditions, QP2 remains confined to the local area underneath the stent and immediately adjacent tissues.

Preclinical data

Both rabbit iliac and porcine coronary models have been utilized in the preclinical evaluations of the QuaDDS-QP2 stent. Doses of 1500 and 3200 μg have been evaluated at 4 and 8 weeks. A significant reduction in neointimal thickening in the absense of thrombus, acute inflammation, fibrosis, foreign body reactions, medial thinning, IEL and EEL disruptions was found. Chronic inflammation was minimal, cellular necrosis was mild to moderate, and the presence of granulation tissue was also minimal.

Clinical data

In the first clinical study (open, randomized, single-center) with the QuaDDS-QP2 stent, 14 QuaDDS-QP2 stents were implanted in 13 patients and 18 control bare QueST stents in 14 patients [Grube et al, 2000, 2001]. Stent sizes were 3.0 and 3.5 mm diameter with stent lengths of 13 mm and 17 mm. After 18 months, the binary restenosis rate in the coated stent group was 0% as compared to 54% in the control group. MACE after 18 months was 0% in the drug stents and 15% in the control group. The 2-year follow-up data showed no binary restenosis with an TLR of 0. Thus, the implantation of the QuaDDS-QP2 stent was extremely efficient with no side-effects (MACE =0). IVUS data revealed only minimal amount of neointimal proliferation [Honda et al, 2001].

The SCORE trial

The SCORE trial (Study to COmpare REstenosis rate between QueST and QuaDDS-QP2) was the first randomized, multicenter trial with the QuaDDS-QP2 stent. The primary endpoint was target vessel revascularization (TVR) with an anticipated reduction in restenosis rate to < 20% as compared to an expected restenosis rate of 24% to 42% seen with traditional stainless steel stents. Sample size calculated to support this goal was 400 patients from 17 sites in Europe and Australia (Principal Investigator: E. Grube). Inclusion criteria were: de novo lesions in native coronary arteries and a narrowing of ≥ 50% and ≤ 100% with reference diameters between ≥ 3.0 mm and ≤ 3.5 mm. Implanted QuaDDS-QP2 stents were either 13 mm or 17 mm long, the target lesion length had to be suitable for stenting with a single Quanam stent. Predilatation before stent implanation was a mandatory part of the protocol, and ticlopidine/clopidogrel was prescribed for 6 months.

Interim analysis of safety outcomes lead to termination of the study. At that time 266 evaluable patients were enrolled (127 drug eluting stent and 139 control). Specifically, there was no stent thrombosis in the control group and a 5.5% stent thrombosis rate present in the QuaDDS-QP2 group (95% confidence interval 3.5–7.5). There was also an increase in periprocedural myocardial infarctions that were usually related to side branch occlusion caused by the polymer bands (although lesions involving a side branch > 2.0 mm was one of the exclusion criteria). MACE at 30 days was 10.2%, predominantly due to subacute stent thrombosis and myocardial infarction. The events could not be attributed to a single underlying cause including protocol violations (like absence of predilatation). The duration of treatment with ticlopidine/clopidogrel was extended from 6 months to 1 year in patients with the active stent.

A full interim evaluation of 6 month angiographic results and clinical efficacy is underway with planned results in November 2001. Nevertheless, interim results from the IVUS substudy show that of the patients evaluated at follow-up (54 QuaDDS-QP2 and 52 controls) there were no significant differences in baseline IVUS parameters including stent expansion. There were promising and significant decreases at follow-up in MLA loss and neointimal area consistent with a reduction in neointima formation.

Upcoming clinical trials

For the time being, no further studies are planned with the QuaDDS-QP2 stent.

Future aspects

The preliminary data from the SCORE trial demonstrate the proof of principle for stents coated with antiproliferative drugs. It also points to the need for diligent preclinical dosing studies to minimize the potential for both acute and subacute events. Because of the similar histological changes observed with both brachytherapy and taxol-eluting stents a more aggressive use of antiplatelet therapy seems mandatory after both treatments [Silber *et al.* 2001].

References

1. Grube E, Gerckens U, Rowold S, Yeung AC, Stertzer SH. Inhibition of in-stent restenosis by a drug eluting polymer stent: pilot trial with 18 month follow-up. *Circulation* 2000;**102**:II–554.

2. Honda Y, Grube E, de la Fuente LM, Yock PG, Stertzer SH, Fitzgerald PJ. Novel drug delivery stent: intravascular ultrasound observations from the first human experience with the QP2-eluting polymer stent system. *Circulation* 2001; **104**: 380–3.

3. Honda Y, Grube E, de la Fuente LM, Yock PG, Fitzgerald PJ, Stertzer SH. A novel drug-delivery stent: intravascular ultrasound observations from the first human experience with the QUANAM QuaDS-QP2 stent system. *J Am Coll Cardiol* 2001;**37**:74A.

4. Kingston DGI. QP2. *Pharmac Ther* 1991;**52**:1–34.

5. Silber S, Brockhoff C, Doerr R, Mügge A, Krischke I, v. Rottkay P, Meinertz T: The German IST-Registry: Need of one year of clopidogrel to avoid late/late stent thrombosis. *J Am Coll Cardiol* 2001;**37**:82A.

42. THE SIROLIMUS-ELUTING BX VELOCITY™ STENT: PRECLINICAL DATA

Andrew J Carter and Robert Falotico

Rationale

The long-term clinical efficacy of intracoronary stenting is limited by restenosis, which occurs in 15 to 30% of patients.[1,2] In-stent restenosis is due solely to neointimal hyperplasia.[3–5] Stent-induced mechanical arterial injury and a foreign body response to the prosthesis incites acute and chronic inflammation in the vessel wall with elaboration of cytokines and growth factors that induce multiple signaling pathways to activate SMC migration and proliferation.[3–5] Drug eluting stents have been proposed as a means of preventing stent thrombosis and restenosis.[6,7] Immobilized heparin surface coating of stents appears to reduce stent thrombogenicity favorably.[7] The efficacy of drug eluting stents for the prevention of restenosis has been limited by issues of polymer biocompatibility, suitability of pharmacological agents, suboptimal in vivo pharmacokinetic properties and local drug toxicity.[6,8]

Experimental data suggest that inhibition of cell cycle progression with prolonged parenteral sirolimus (SRL) may be an effective strategy to prevent restenosis.[8–10] SRL is a potent immunosuppressive agent with anti-inflammatory and antiproliferative effects. Gallo et al. recently demonstrated a reduction in post-angioplasty restenosis with prolonged systemic SRL therapy in a porcine coronary model of restenosis.[10] SRL is a hydrophobic drug that has low solubility in aqueous solutions.[11,12] Because of its lipophilicity, the drug passes easily through cell membranes, enabling intramural distribution and prolonged arterial tissue retention.[12] Further, cellular uptake is enhanced by binding to the cytosolic receptor, FKBP 12, which also may enhance chronic tissue retention of SRL. Thus, the known biologic effects and pharmacokinetic properties of SRL suggest that the agent is an ideal candidate for a stent-based delivery to prevent restenosis.

Polymer and drug-eluting stents

Long stainless steel balloon expandable tubular stents (18 mm) (Cordis Co, Warren, NJ) are coated with a thin layer (10 μm) of a non-erodable methacrylate and ethylene-based co-polymer containing approximately 185 μg of SRL (Wyeth-Ayerst, Princeton, NJ) by weight. The total drug and polymer weight is approximately 500 μg and the ratio of drug to polymer is approximately 30% for the SRL-eluting stent.

Molecular action of sirolimus

Gregory *et al.* demonstrated that intraperitoneal administration of SRL, a potent immunosuppressive agent, resulted in a dose-dependent inhibition of arterial intimal thickening caused by either chronic alloimmune or mechanical injury in a rat model.[13] Subsequent studies by Marx *et al.* reported that SRL inhibited both human and rat VSMC proliferation in vitro by blocking G_1/S transition.[14,15] The inhibition of proliferation was mediated by SRL binding to its cytosolic receptor, FKBP12, and associated with reduced cdk2 activity and pRb phosphorylation. Gallo *et al.* recently demonstrated that systemic SRL therapy significantly reduces the proliferative response after coronary angioplasty in the porcine model.[10] The antiproliferative effects of SRL after PTCA were attributed to an inhibition of the pRB phosphorylation and preventing the downregulation of p27[kip1]. Thus, the antiproliferative activity of SRL after balloon arterial injury in conjunction with its immunosuppressive properties suggests that this drug could also be useful for the prevention of in-stent restenosis.

In vivo pharmacokinetics

In vivo pharmacokinetic studies in the porcine coronary model demonstrated that the whole blood concentration of SRL peaked at 1 hour (2.63 ± 0.74 ng/ml) after stent deployment and then declined below the lower limit of detection (0.4 ng/ml) by 3 days. The total arterial tissue level of SRL was 97 ± 13 ng/artery and the residual stent content was 71 ± 10 µg at 3 days. The amount of residual SRL on the stent at 3 days was 43% of the initial quantity loaded on the stent. A modification of the coating has provided similar arterial tissue levels at 28 days as compared with 3 days for the present drug coating. These data document the ability to deliver and achieve a potentially therapeutic arterial tissue concentration of SRL in the porcine model and insignificant levels in the systemic circulation using the non-erodable methacrylate and ethylene-based co-polymer matrix.

Preclinical efficacy studies

Preclinical efficacy studies demonstrated a 35 to 50% reduction in in-stent neointimal hyperplasia for the SRL-eluting stents as compared with bare metal stents at 28 days in the porcine and rabbit model (Table 42.1). We recently completed an experimental study in the porcine coronary model comparing bare metal, dexamethasone (DEX), SRL and a combination of DEX + SRL

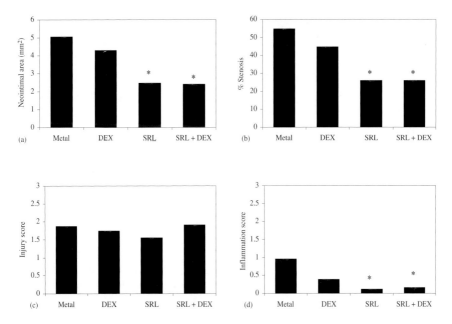

Figure 42.1: *Bar graphs demonstrate a significant reduction in neointimal area (a) and per cent in-stent stenosis (b) for SRL coated as compared with the bare metal stents. Strut induced arterial injury is similar for each stent group (c), while the extent of strut-associated inflammation is reduced in arteries containing DEX or SRL-eluting stents (d). (*P <0.0001 versus metal, †P = 0.09 versus metal, ‡P = 0.002 versus metal.)*

coated stents. The mean vessel injury scores were similar for the drug coated and metal control stents (Figure 42.1). The DEX- and SRL-eluting stents had significantly lower strut-associated inflammation scores as compared with the bare metal stents . Strut-associated inflammation was significantly reduced for the SRL (0.13 ± 0.34) as compared with metal stents (0.97 ± 1.10, $P <0.0001$). Stent-based delivery of SRL alone or combined with DEX resulted in a 50% reduction in neointimal area as compared with bare metal stents, whereas DEX alone had a modest and non-significant effect on neointimal formation. The mean neointimal area was 2.47 ± 1.04 mm^2 for the SRL alone, and 2.42 ± 1.04 mm^2 for the SRL and DEX as compared with the metal (5.06 ± 1.88 mm^2, $P <0.0001$) or DEX coated stents (4.31 ± 3.21 mm^2, $P < 0.001$). Thus, the per cent area stenosis was significantly less for the SRL (24 ± 10%) and the SRL + DEX (24 ± 13%) as compared with bare metal (47 ± 19%, $P <0.0001$) or DEX coated stents (45 ± 31%, $P <0.001$).

Table 42.1: Summary of histologic data at 28 days after placement of control and drug-eluting stents in porcine coronary arteries

Group	Vessel area (MM²)	Neointimal area (mm²)	% Stenosis	Inflammation score	Injury score
Metal (n = 8)	12.72 ± 2.87	5.06 ± 1.08	55 ± 20	0.97 ± 1.09	1.88 ± 1.07
DEX (n = 7)	12.47 ± 2.24	4.31 ± 3.12	45 ± 31‡	0.39 ± 0.50§	1.75 ± 1.04
SRL (n = 8)	12.11± 1.28	2.47±1.04*†	26±11*†	0.12±0.34*	1.56±0.72
SRL + DEX (n = 6)	12.15 ± 1.55	2.42 ± 1.72*†	26 ± 19*†	0.17 ± 0.64*	1.92 ± 0.58

Data is expressed as mean ± SD
* P <0.0001 versus metal
† P < 0.001 versus DEX
‡ P = 0.09 versus metal
§ P = 0.0022 versus metal

An independent blinded histological assessment revealed the presence of typical cellular components of the neointima and a similar degree of endothelialization for the SRL as compared with the bare metal stents. The arterial wall morphology at 28 days for the SRL-eluting and the bare metal stents are illustrated in Figure 42.2. The morphology of non-stented reference

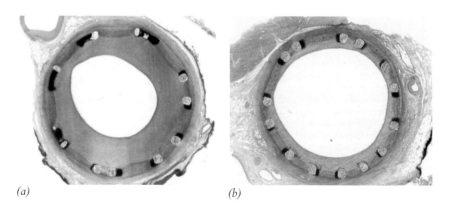

(a)   *(b)*

Figure 42.2: *Low power photomicrographs at 28 days after oversized stent placement in normal porcine coronary arteries. (a) A bare metal stent with moderate neointimal formation encroaching the lumen. (b) The SRL-eluting stent has significantly less neointima as compared with the bare metal stent despite a similar degree of vessel injury. The photomicrograph of the SRL-eluting stent demonstrates minimal neointimal formation consisting of SMC and matrix proteoglycans. (H & E, 2.1 × magnification.)*

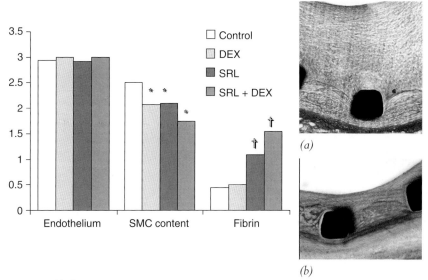

(a)

(b)

Figure 42.3: *The bar graph demonstrates the effects of a bare metal and drug-eluting stents on arterial repair. The SMC content score was less for the drug-eluting stents as compared with the bare metal stents (P <0.0001). Intimal fibrin scores were 2-fold greater for the SRL versus metal stents (P <0.0001), whereas the DEX stents exhibited a similar degree of residual fibrin deposition. The stent endothelialization scores were identical for the metal as compared with sirolimus stents. High power photomicrographs of bare metal (a) and SRL-polymer coated (b) stents demonstrate some of the morphologic features of the arterial wall at 28 days after implant. The neointima of the SRL-eluting stent contains SMC with grade 1 residual fibrin deposition.*

arterial wall sections, including the vessel area, neointimal area and per cent area stenosis, was similar for the metal and each of the drug-eluting stents. The appearance of the neointima was more variable for each of the drug-coated stent groups as compared with the bare metal stents. In general, the neointima of the SRL-coated stents consisted of SMC, matrix proteoglycans and scant focal regions of residual fibrin adjacent to the stent struts (Figure 42.3). Focal medial necrosis or intimal hemorrhage was not observed within any of the bare metal or drug-coated stents.

A semi-quantitative histological grading system demonstrated less SMC colonization and more residual fibrin deposition for the sirolimus-eluting stents as compared with the bare metal stents (Figure 42.3). The SMC content score was less for the drug-eluting stents as compared with the bare metal stents (metal, 2.09 ± 0.30 versus SRL, 2.50 ± 0.51, $P = 0.002$). Intimal fibrin scores were higher for the SRL (1.09 ± 0.73) versus metal

A   St   SRL Dex

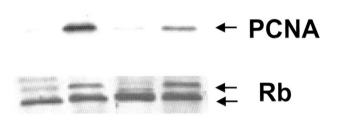

← PCNA

⇇ Rb

Figure 42.4: *Representative Western blots demonstrating the effect of an SRL-coated stent on cellular proliferation, phosphorylation of pRb, and inflammatory cytokine production at 7 days as shown by a reduction in PCNA and an increase in hypophosphorylated pRb versus the hyperphosphorylated (ppRb) form of the retinoblastoma protein.*

stents (0.44 ± 0.56 P <0.0001), whereas the DEX stents exhibited a similar degree of residual fibrin deposition (0.50 ± 0.69). Endothelialization scores were identical for the metal (2.9 ± 0.4) as compared with SRL stents (2.9 ± 0.4, P = 0.66). Therefore, critical reparative events, such as endothelialization and SMC colonization of the neointima, with SRL-eluting stents occurs in a similar temporal sequence as observed with bare metal stents. The focal remnants of residual fibrin deposition observed in the vessels with SRL-coated stents may reflect a delay in arterial repair or impaired fibrin degradation secondary to the local effects of the drug. Long-term studies are required to elucidate if the drug is simply delaying the formation of neointima or subtly impairing fibrin degradation without late neointimal formation.

An analysis of arterial wall protein expression at 7 days was completed to determine the mechanism of action by which stent-based delivery of SRL reduces in-stent neointimal hyperplasia. Western blot analysis demonstrated a profound reduction in PCNA expression in the vessel wall at 7 days for the SRL eluting as compared with bare metal stents (Figure 42.4). We also documented reduced phosphorylation of pRb protein by an SRL-eluting stent, which is consistent with the proven effects of the agent on cell cycle signaling and proliferation. Further, a significant reduction in strut-associated inflammation was observed at 28 days for the SRL as compared with bare metal stents, suggesting the potential for additional mechanisms of action to inhibit neointimal hyperplasia. Analysis of the vessel wall protein expression documented a 70% reduction in the inflammatory cytokine MCP-1 for the SRL-eluting as compared with a bare metal stent. Unlike cyclosporine and

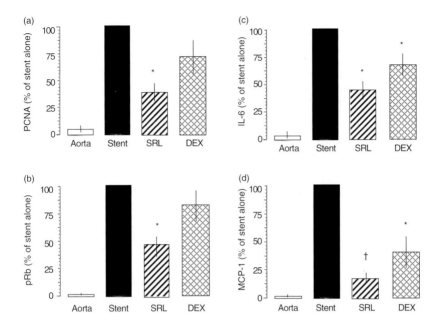

Figure 42.5: Bar graphs summarizing the densitometric analysis of Western blots. Stent placement was associated with increased expression of the cellular proliferation markers PCNA and pRb. These markers of cellular proliferation were reduced by the SRL-eluting stents. The arterial response to stent injury was also associated with enhanced production of the inflammatory cytokines MCP-1 and IL-6. Exposure of vessels to stents coated with either SRL or DEX resulted in lower expression of MCP-1 and IL-6. Data are expressed as mean ± SEM of four separate experiments. (†P <0.01; *P <0.05.)

tacrolimus, SRL is a weak inhibitor of cytokine production. The potent immunosuppressive effect of SRL is directed toward inhibiting the proliferation of T-cells by blocking IL-2 activation of p70[s6] kinase.[12] The observed reduction of MCP-1, in the present study, may be secondary to the effects of SRL on cellular proliferation and the production of cytokines by activated SMC.

Clinical data

The safety and feasibility of an SRL-eluting BX Velocity stent was evaluated in a phase I clinical trial. Thirty patients with stable angina were electively treated with two different formulations of SRL-coated stents. Fifteen patients received a fast release formulation (<15–day drug release) and 15 received a slow release formulation (>28–day drug release). Stent deployment was successful in all cases without in-hospital major adverse cardiac events. Clinical follow-up was obtained after 8 months. Independent quantitative analysis of coronary angiography and intravascular ultrasound immediately after the procedure and at 4 months documented minimal per cent neointimal hyperplasia volume in both groups (11 ± 3.0%, slow release; 10.4 ± 3.0%, fast release).[20] In-lesion late lumen loss was 0.16 ± 0.3 mm (slow release) and −0.1 ± 0.3 mm (fast release). There were no cases of in-stent, in-lesion or edge restenosis. All 30 patients completed 8 months clinical follow-up without a major adverse clinical event (death, myocardial infarction, revascularization, stent thrombosis). These encouraging phase I clinical results substantiated the need for confirmation by placebo-controlled, multicenter clinical trials.

Upcoming clinical trials

The RAndomized study with the sirolimus-eluting Bx VELOCITY balloon expandable stent in the treatment of patients with de novo native coronary Lesions (RAVEL) is a multicenter, prospective, randomized double clinical trial comparing bare metal and the drug-eluting stent. Two hundred and thirty-seven patients will be randomized to a single sirolimus-coated (140 µg/cm^2) versus the metal Bx VELOCITY stent. The primary clinical endpoints are target lesion revascularization and angiographic restenosis at 6 months. Spectacular results were presented at the XXIII Congress of the European Society of Cardiology in Stockholm, September 2001. A zero percent restenosis rate was found in the sirolimus-eluting group versus 26% in the control group. Late loss was −0.01 mm in the sirolimus group and 0.8 mm in the control group at 6 months repeat angiography. Preliminary clinical data showed 26 revascularizations at 6 months in the control group vs 0 in the sirolimus group.

The SIRIUS study is a multicenter, prospective, randomized double blind trial that will be conducted in 55 centers in the United States. Eleven hundred patients with focal de novo native coronary arterial lesions (2.50 to 3.5 mm diameter, 15 mm to 30 mm long) will be randomized to treatment with sirolimus-eluting (109 µg/cm^2) or bare metal Bx VELOCITY balloon expandable stents. The primary endpoints of the SIRIUS trial are target vessel failure (death, myocardial infarction, target lesion revascularization) at 9 months. In addition, secondary endpoints are core laboratory analysis of angiographic and intravascular ultrasound data to determine treatment effects on neointimal hyperplasia and in-stent restenosis. Clinical follow-up will extend to 5 years in order to assess for late events. The enrolment in this trial began in July 2001 and completion of this phase is expected by April 2001. In addition to the pivotal RAVEL and SIRIUS trials, feasibility studies are ongoing to assess efficacy of sirolimus-eluting stents in more complex lesion subset such as in-stent restenosis.

The future

Preclinical and early clinical data provide sufficient evidence to conclude that stent-based delivery of SRL via a non-erodable polymer matrix is feasible and effectively reduces in-stent neointimal hyperplasia. Local stent-based delivery of SRL profoundly suppresses neointimal proliferation and the foreign-body response by inhibiting cell cycle progression and expression of inflammatory cytokines. This novel strategy to prevent restenosis warrants further study to more clearly define the dose response and confirm the biological efficacy in placebo-controlled clinical trials.

References

1. Williams DO, Holubkov R, Yeh W *et al.* Percutaneous coronary interventions in the current era compared with 1985–1986: The National Heart, Lung, and Blood Institute Registries. *Circulation* 2000; **102**:2945–51.

2. Mehran R, Dangas G, Mintz GS *et al.* Patterns of in-stent restenosis: angiographic classification and implications for long-term clinical outcome. *Circulation* 1999; **100**:1872–8.

3. Farb A, Sangiorgi G, Carter AJ *et al.* Pathology of acute and chronic coronary stenting in humans. *Circulation* 1999; **99**:44–52.

4. Grewe P, Deneke T, Machraoui A. Acute and chronic tissue response to coronary stent implantation: pathologic findings in human specimen. *J Am Coll Cardiol* 2000; **35**:157–63.

5. Kornowski R, Hong MK, Tio FO *et al.* In-stent restenosis: contributions of inflammatory responses and arterial injury to neointimal hyperplasia. *J Am Coll Cardiol* 1998; **31**:224–30.

6. Bertrand OF, Sipehia R, Mongrain R, Rodes J, Tardif JC, Bilodeau L, Cote G, Bourassa MG. Biocompatibility aspects of new stent technology. *J Am Coll Cardiol* 1998; **32**:562–71.

7. Hårdhammar PA, van Beusekom HMM, Emanuelsson HU et al. Reduction in

thrombotic events with heparin-coated Palmaz-Schatz stents in normal porcine coronary arteries. *Circulation* 1996; **93**:423–30.

8. Topol EJ, Serruys PW. Frontiers in interventional cardiology. *Circulation.* 1998; **98**:1802–20.

9. Braun-Dullaeus RC, Mann MJ, Dzau VJ. Cell cycle progression: new therapeutic target for vascular proliferative disease. *Circulation* 1998; **98**:82–9.

10. Gallo R, Padurean A, Jayaraman T *et al*. Inhibition of intimal thickening after balloon angioplasty in porcine coronary arteries by targeting regulators of the cell cycle. *Circulation* 1999; **99**:2164–70.

11. Gummert JF, Ikonen T, Morris RE. Newer immunosuppressive drugs: a review. *J Am Soc Nephrol* 1999; **10**:1366–80.

12. Schreiber S. Chemistry and biology of the immunophilins and their immunosuppressive ligands. *Science* 1991; **251**:283–7.

13. Gregory CR, Huie P, Billingham ME, Morris RE. Rapamycin inhibits arterial intimal thickening caused by both alloimmune and mechanical injury. *Transplantation* 1993; **55**:1409–18.

14. Poon M, Marx SO, Gallo R *et al*. Rapamycin inhibits VSMC migration. *J Clin Invest* 1996; **98**:2277–83.

15. Marx SO, Jayaraman T, Go LO, Marks AR. Rapamycin-FKBP inhibits cell cycle regulators of proliferation in VSMC. *Circ Res* 1995; **76**:412–17.

16. Carter AJ, Wilensky R, Bailey LR *et al*. Stent-based sirolimus therapy reduces neointimal formation and in-stent restenosis in a porcine coronary model . *J Am Coll Cardiol* 2000; **35**:13A (abstract).

17. Suzuki T, Bailey LR, Kopia G *et al*. Synergistic efficacy of anti-proliferative and anti-inflammatory therapies delivered by a stent. *Circulation* 2000; **102**:II-566 (abstract).

18. Carter AJ, Kopia G, Bailey LR *et al*. Temporal effects on arterial repair of a sustained release formulation of sirolimus eluting from a stent. *J Am Coll Cardiol* 2001; **37**:1A (abstract).

19. Klugherz BD, Llanos G, Lieuallen W *et al*. Stent-based delivery of sirolimus for the prevention of restenosis. *J Am Coll Cardiol* 2000; **35**:58A (abstract).

20. Sousa JE, Costa M, Abizaid AC *et al*. Lack of neointimal proliferation after implantation of sirolimus-coated stents in human coronary arteries: a quantitative coronary angiography and three-dimensional intravascular ultrasound study. *Circulation* 2000; **102**:r54–r57.

43. THE SIROLIMUS-ELUTING Bx VELOCITY™ STENT: CLINICAL DATA

Marco A Costa and J Eduardo Sousa

Rationale

A number of systemic antiproliferative approaches to reduce restenosis after angioplasty have been tested, but promising results from experimental laboratories have not been translated into clinical effectiveness.[1] The failure to achieve adequate drug concentrations in the target coronary segment is the major drawback of systemic antirestenotic drug therapy. Local drug delivery systems have been proposed to overcome this problem. Clinical experience with microporous, hydrogel balloons, iontophoretic catheters, dispatch catheters and infusion sleeves has been reported.[2–6] However, the rapid washout of the drug downstream into the coronary circulation decreases the amount of agent actually deposited within the arterial wall to <5%.[2,7] As a result of their permanent scaffolding action, stents have become the most attractive reservoir for sustained delivery of intramural antiproliferative agents. A prolonged and sufficient local drug concentration may be achieved via drug-eluting stents a novel antirestenotic technology recently introduced into the clinical arena.

Molecular action of Sirolimus

Sirolimus (rapamycin, Rapamune®), the antiproliferative agent applied onto the surface of the Bx VELOCITY™ stent (Cordis, Warren, NJ), is a natural macrocyclic lactone with potent immunosuppressive effect. It was developed by Wyeth-Ayerst Laboratories and approved by the Food and Drug Administration (FDA) for the prophylaxis of renal transplant rejection in 1999. Similar to cyclosporin A and tacrolimus (FK506), sirolimus binds to specific cytosolic proteins, the so-called immunophilins. However, the sirolimus:FKBP complex does not affect calcineurin activity. The mechanism of action of sirolimus is distinct from other immunosuppressive agents that act solely by inhibiting DNA synthesis. The sirolimus:FKBP complex binds to a specific cell cycle regulatory protein, the mTOR (mammalian target of rapamycin), and inhibits its activation. The inhibition of mTOR elicits a number of important effects: inhibition of translation of a family of mRNAs

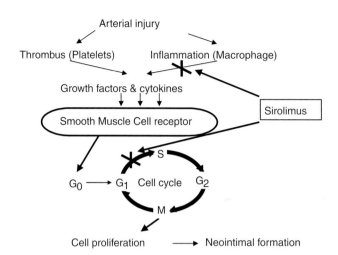

Figure 43.1:
Schematic illustration of the mechanism of action of Sirolimus.

that code for proteins essential for cell cycle progression, elevation of p27 levels leading to inhibition of cyclin/CDK complexes and ultimately induction of cell cycle arrest in late G1 phase (Figure 43.1).[8–10] The upregulation of FK506-binding protein 12 (FKBP12) observed in neointimal human smooth muscle cells further supports the potential antirestenotic effect of rapamycin.[11] Its low toxicity[12] and potent cytostatic action place sirolimus high on the list of antirestenotic agents for local drug delivery.

Drug–polymer matrix and elution kinetics

Sirolimus was blended in a 50:50 mixture of non-erodable polymers that have been used clinically in bone cements, ocular devices, and in a drug-releasing intrauterine device.[13,14] Both synthetic polymers have the ability to expand uniformly with the stent and maintain its smoothness and chemical characteristics after sterilization (Figure 43.2).

A 5 μm thick layer of sirolimus–polymer matrix was applied onto the surface of the Bx VELOCITY™ stent, a laser cut 316L stainless steel balloon expandable stent (Cordis, Warren, NJ). In vivo experiments have shown that sirolimus levels in whole blood peak at 1 hour (2.6 ± 0.7 ng/ml – fast release coating; 0.9 ng/ml $\pm$ 0.2 ng/ml – slow release coating) after implantation and fall below the lower limit of quantification by 72 hours (0.4 ng/ml).[15] Taking into account that renal transplant patients maintain chronic blood levels of rapamycin between 8 and 17 ng/ml, the peak blood level after implantation of the sirolimus-coated stent is absolutely negligible.

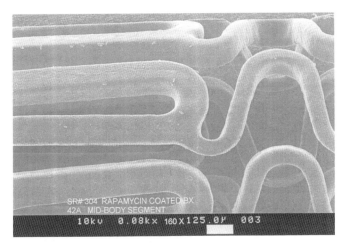

Figure 43.2: *Scanning electron microscope image of Sirolimus-eluting Bx VELOCITY*™ *stent.*

The drug is almost completely eluted by 15 days after implantation (fast release formulation). To prolong the drug release rate to >28 days (slow release formulation), another layer of drug-free polymer was applied onto the top of the drug–polymer matrix, introducing a diffusion barrier. The Bx VELOCITY™ stents, regardless of the coating formulation, were loaded with a fixed amount of sirolimus per unit of metal surface area (140 μg sirolimus/cm²).

Preclinical data

In vitro studies have demonstrated the ability of rapamycin to inhibit proliferation of both rat and human smooth muscle cells.[10,16,17] Thus, systemic administration of sirolimus has been tested to reduce intimal thickening in models of vascular injury.[9,18–20] Gregory *et al.* first reported the antirestenotic effect of rapamycin in vivo. In rat carotid arteries, 1.5 mg/kg per day of rapamycin given from day 0 to 13 after balloon injury reduced intimal thickening by 45% and substantially decreased macrophage infiltration compared to control.[18] Gallo *et al.* reported the efficacy of systemic administration of rapamycin in reducing neointimal hyperplasia in a porcine model of restenosis. Intramuscular administration of rapamycin, started 3 days before PTCA at a dose of 0.5 mg/kg and continued for 14 days at a dose of 0.25 mg/kg, was associated with >40% reduction in coronary stenosis after balloon angioplasty.[9]

Carter *et al.* implanted sirolimus-eluting Bx VELOCITY™ stents in a porcine restenosis model.[21] While a similar degree of re-endothelialization was observed in both drug-eluting and bare stents, neointimal proliferation was markedly reduced by rapamycin-coated stents. Recently, the same group has demonstrated a reduced strut associated inflammation and increased intimal fibrin scores after implantation of sirolimus-eluting stent as compared with metal stents.[22] Klugherz *et al.* tested the effectiveness of sirolimus-eluting stents in rabbit iliac arteries. Again, drug-coated stents showed a 23–45% reduction in neointimal proliferation compared to both bare and polymer coated stents.[15]

Clinical data

As a result of these promising experimental observations, a pilot clinical study was initiated to test the feasibility of the sirolimus-eluting Bx VELOCITY™ stent in humans. Our group first performed the implantation of a sirolimus-coated stent in human coronary arteries.[23] Thirty patients with angina pectoris were electively treated with two different formulations of sirolimus-coated stents (slow release [SR], $n = 15$ and fast release [FR], $n = 15$). Four months

Table 43.1: Comparison between sirolimus-eluting Bx VELOCITY™ stent and other stent technologies

Stent	Length (mm)	IVUS – NIH (mm³) 4–6 month angiography	I year
Multilink (bare)*	22.2	46.0 ± 31.9	—
NIR (bare)*	18.5	39.9 ± 27.6	—
Bx VELOCITY (bare)	18.0	39.01 ± 21.5	—
Radioactive	15.0	18.6 ± 12.5	27.7 ± 11.9
Bx VELOCITY	18.0	0.4 ± 0.93	3.2± 2.4
(Rapamycin)§			

* Costa *et al., Am J Cardiol* 2000; 85:135
† Feres *et al,. ACC,* 2001.
‡ Kay *et al., Circulation,* 2001; 103:34.
§ Sousa *et al., ACC,* 2001.
IVUS = Intravascular ultrasound
NIH = Neointimal hyperplasia

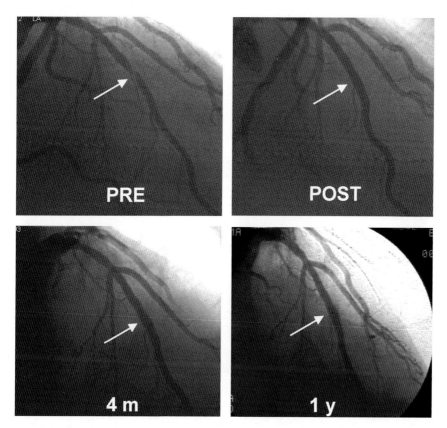

Figure 43.3: *Angiography shows a lesion in the mid-portion of the left anterior descending coronary (white arrow), which was treated with the implantation of a sirolimus-coated Bx VELOCITY™ stent (upper, right panel). Lumen dimensions were maintained at 4- and 12-month follow-up (lower panels).*

later, there was minimal neointimal hyperplasia in both groups by intravascular ultrasound (IVUS) or quantitative coronary angiography (in-stent late loss = 0.09 mm ± 0.3 mm [SR] and –0.02 mm ± 0.3 mm [FR]; in-lesion late loss = 0.16 mm ± 0.3 mm [SR] and –0.1 mm ± 0.3 mm [FR]).[23] No in-stent or edge restenosis (diameter stenosis ≥50%) was observed. Rensing *et al.* have also implanted 15 slow release rapamycin-coated Bx VELOCITY™ stents in human coronary arteries at the Thoraxcenter, Rotterdam.[24] One patient died due to cerebral bleeding and 13 patients returned for 6–month follow-up. None had angiographic restenosis or any cardiac event. In-stent neointimal hyperplasia was also minimal at 6–month volumetric 3D-IVUS analysis. One-year follow-up of the 30 patients treated in Brazil has been recently reported.[25] No major clinical event (thrombosis, repeat revascularization, myocardial infarction or death) occurred up to 12 months. Again, minimal neointimal proliferation was observed by IVUS (Table 43.1) or angiography (Figure 43.3), demonstrating a sustained suppression of neointimal proliferation in this first series of patients treated with sirolimus-eluting stent.[25] Eighteen-month angiographic and IVUS follow-up of the patients treated in Holland is planned.

Upcoming trials

Two multicenter randomized trials are already underway. The RAVEL trial enrolled 220 patients with de novo coronary stenosis in 18 Latin American and European centers. Patients were randomized to receive either a Sirolimus-eluting Bx VELOCITY™ stent or a bare metal Bx VELOCITY™ stent. The primary end-point is late loss in minimal lumen diameter at 6-month angiography. Spectacular results were presented at the XXIII Congress of the European Society of Cardiology in Stockholm, September 2001. A zero percent restenosis rate was found in the sirolimus-eluting group versus 26% in the control group. Late loss was –0.01 mm in the sirolimus group and 0.8 mm in the control group at 6 months repeat angiography. Preliminary clinical data showed 26 revascularizations at 6 months in the control group vs 0 in the sirolimus group.. The US randomized study (SIRIUS trial) has started, and will enrol 1100 patients with de novo coronary lesions in 50 centers. Results are expected in 2002.

Future directions

Whether sirolimus-eluting Bx VELOCITY™ stents represent a turning point in the treatment of coronary artery disease will be determined only after the results of the upcoming large randomized clinical trials, but results from the pilot studies are already very encouraging. The next step will be the application of this new technology for the treatment of more complex situations such as: in-stent restenosis, ostial and bifurcated lesions, long lesions, total occlusions, saphenous vein grafts, small vessels, main stem stenosis, multivessel disease, in the setting of acute myocardial infarction, peripheral disease, diabetic patients, etc. A pilot investigation testing the feasibility and efficacy of the sirolimus-eluting Bx VELOCITY™ stent for the treatment of in-stent restenosis is already underway at the Institute Dante Pazzanese of Cardiology in Brazil and at the Thoraxcenter in The Netherlands. Results will be available by the end of 2001.

References

1. Lafont A, Faxon D. Why do animal models of post-angioplasty restenosis sometimes poorly predict the outcome of clinical trials? *Cardiovasc Res* 1998; **39**:50–9.

2. Camenzind E, Kutryk MJ, Serruys PW. Use of locally delivered conventional drug therapies. *Semin Interv Cardiol* 1996; **1**:67–76.

3. Mitchel JF, Fram DB, Palme DF, II *et al.* Enhanced intracoronary thrombolysis with urokinase using a novel, local drug delivery system. In vitro, in vivo, and clinical studies. *Circulation* 1995; **91**:785–93.

4. Kornowski R, Hong MK, Tio FO *et al.* A randomized animal study evaluating the efficacies of locally delivered heparin and urokinase for reducing in-stent restenosis. *Coronary Art Dis* 1997; **8**:293–8.

5. Bartorelli AL, De Cesare NB, Kaplan AV *et al.* Local heparin delivery prior to coronary stent implantation: acute and six-month clinical and angiographic results. *Cathet Cardiovasc Diagn* 1997; **42**:313–20.

6. Robinson KA, Chronos NA, Schieffer E *et al.* Endoluminal local delivery of PCNA/cdc2 antisense oligonucleotides by porous balloon catheter does not affect neointima formation or vessel size in the pig coronary artery model of postangioplasty restenosis. *Cathet Cardiovasc Diagn* 1997; **41**:348–53.

7. Lincoff AM, Topol EJ, Ellis SG. Local drug delivery for the prevention of restenosis. Fact, fancy, and future. *Circulation* 1994; **90**:2070–84.

8. Roque M, Cordon-Cardo C, Fuster V *et al.* Modulation of apoptosis, proliferation, and p27 expression in a porcine coronary angioplasty model. *Atherosclerosis* 2000; **153**:315–22.

9. Gallo R, Padurean A, Jayaraman T *et al.* Inhibition of intimal thickening after balloon angioplasty in porcine coronary arteries by targeting regulators of the cell cycle. *Circulation* 1999; **99**:2164–70.

10. Marx SO, Jayaraman T, Go LO *et al.* Rapamycin-FKBP inhibits cell cycle regulators of proliferation in vascular smooth muscle cells. *Circ Res* 1995; **76**:412–17.

11. Zohlnhofer D, Klein CA, Richter T *et al.* Gene expression profiling of human stent-induced neointima by cDNA array analysis of microscopic specimens retrieved by helix cutter atherectomy: detection of FK506-binding protein 12 upregulation. *Circulation* 2001; **103**:1396–402.

12. Groth CG, Backman L, Morales JM *et al.* Sirolimus (rapamycin)-based therapy in human renal transplantation: similar efficacy and different toxicity compared with cyclosporine. Sirolimus European Renal Transplant Study Group. *Transplantation* 1999; **67**:1036–42.

13. Kindt-Larsen T, Smith DB, Jensen JS. Innovations in acrylic bone cement and application equipment. *J Appl Biomat* 1995; **6**:75–83.

14. Revell PA, Braden M, Freeman MA. Review of the biological response to a novel bone cement containing poly(ethyl methacrylate) and *n*-butyl methacrylate. *Biomaterials* 1998; **19**:1579–86.

15. Klugherz B, Llanos G, Lieuallen W *et al*. *J Am Coll Cardiol* 2000; **35**:58A (Abstract).

16. Mohacsi PJ, Tuller D, Hulliger B *et al*. Different inhibitory effects of immunosuppressive drugs on human and rat aortic smooth muscle and endothelial cell proliferation stimulated by platelet-derived growth factor or endothelial cell growth factor. *J Heart Lung Transpl* 1997; **16**:484–92.

17. Poon M, Marx SO, Gallo R *et al*. Rapamycin inhibits vascular smooth muscle cell migration. *J Clin Invest* 1996; **98**:2277–83.

18. Gregory CR, Huie P, Billingham ME *et al*. Rapamycin inhibits arterial intimal thickening caused by both alloimmune and mechanical injury. Its effect on cellular, growth factor, and cytokine response in injured vessels. *Transplantation* 1993; **55**:1409–18.

19. Gregory CR, Huang X, Pratt RE *et al*. Treatment with rapamycin and mycophenolic acid reduces arterial intimal thickening produced by mechanical injury and allows endothelial replacement. *Transplantation* 1995; **59**:655–61.

20. Burke SE, Lubbers NL, Chen YW *et al*. Neointimal formation after balloon-induced vascular injury in Yucatan minipigs is reduced by oral rapamycin. *J Cardiovasc Pharmacol* 1999; **33**:829–35.

21. Carter A, Bailey L, Llanos G *et al*. *J Am Coll Cardiol* 2000; **35**:13A.

22. Suzuki T, Kopia G, Bailey L *et al*. Experimental results with a sirolimus eluting stent: a comprehensive histological analysis. *J Am Coll Cardiol* 2001; **37**:1A-648A.

23. Sousa JE, Costa MA, Abizaid A *et al*. Lack of neointimal proliferation after implantation of sirolimus-coated stents in human coronary arteries: a quantitative coronary angiography and three-dimensional intravascular ultrasound study. *Circulation* 2001; **103**:192–5.

24. Rensing B, Vos J, Smits P *et al*. Coronary restenosis prevention with a rapamycin coated stent. *J Am Coll Cardiol* 2001; **37**:1A-648A.

25. Sousa JEMR, Costa MA, Abizaid A *et al*. Mid-(4-Month) and long-term (1-Year) QCA and three-dimensional IVUS follow-up after implantation of sirolimus-coated stent in human coronary arteries. *J Am Coll Cardiol* 2001; **37**:1A-648A.